FIGHT YOUR PHOBIA
– AND WIN

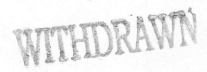

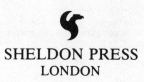

SHELDON PRESS
LONDON

First published in Great Britain in 1984 by
Sheldon Press, Marylebone Road, London NW1 4DU

Fourth impression 1991

British Library Cataloguing in Publication Data

Lewis, David
    Fight your phobia and win.—(Overcoming common
    problems)
    1. Phobias
    I. Title   II. Series
    616.85′225068   RC535

    ISBN 0–85969–398–8

Filmset by Inforum Ltd, Portsmouth
and printed in Great Britain at the
University Press, Cambridge

FIGHT YOUR PHOBIA – AND WIN

DAVID LEWIS is a research and clinical psychologist, and is currently carrying out research funded by the Medical Research Council at Sussex University. He lectures widely in Britain and overseas, and is the clinical director of 'Stresswatch'. He has written a number of books on aspects of psychology, especially on anxiety and on intelligence, and is co-author of *Thrive on Stress* and *The Anxiety Antidote*, and author of *Fit Kit*, also published by Sheldon Press.

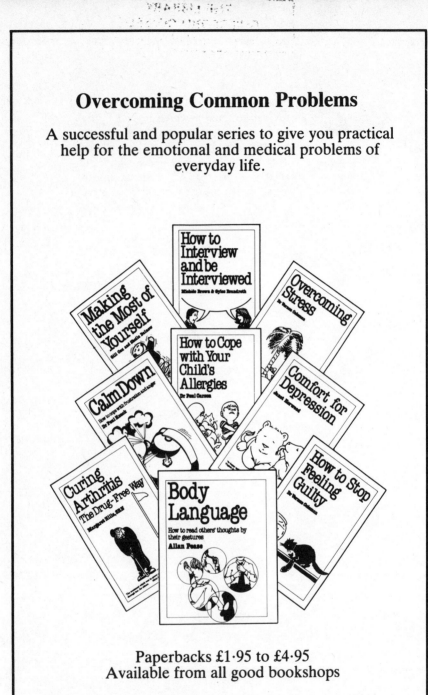

To Dr Keith Oatley,
with my grateful thanks for his advice
and encouragement.

Contents

How to Use This Book

Because this is a practical book designed to teach you important and powerful psychological skills, it is necessary to read each part in the right order.

In Part One I will explain what phobias are as well as how and why they develop. We will be looking at common misconceptions about the nature of phobias and you will learn why telling yourself not to be so 'silly' may only make you feel even more fearful. You will learn how the mental and physical symptoms of anxiety arise, and what puts some people at greater risk of phobias than others.

This knowledge provides the essential background against which you can start work with the practical procedures detailed in the self-help programme. You will need the understanding and insights which Part One offers before moving on to the actual training, so please do not feel tempted to skip ahead.

The six-step programme in Part Two teaches all the procedures necessary for creating a self-help programme which matches your personal needs. By using these procedures in the way described you should be able to overcome any type of phobia.

Please work through each of the stages carefully and only move on once you have completed all the tasks and mastered the procedures described.

Part One

1

Understanding Your Phobia

Many millions of perfectly healthy men, women and children are made extremely frightened by things which other people see no reason to fear. This type of acute anxiety is called a *phobia* from the Greek word *phobos* meaning a 'dread' or 'horror'. Because the fears seem so irrational and unreasonable it is often difficult for non-phobics either to understand a sufferer's feelings or to sympathize with his, or her, problems.

The hidden fear

As a result, phobias are frequently hidden fears, carefully concealed by those who suffer from them, from friends, neighbours or colleagues at work and sometimes even from members of their own family. Ashamed of what they regard as 'foolish' feelings, dreading ridicule, and sometimes embarrassed by what they are convinced is a form of serious mental illness, a vast number of phobics endure their anguish in silence and in secret.

Often their distress is increased by feelings of depression and guilt. They are sad because anxiety has restricted their lives, preventing them from doing things they used to enjoy and depriving them of the pleasures most people take for granted. They may also feel guilty about the effects, real or imagined, which their phobia is having on those they love. They often see themselves as failures who have let down their spouse and ruined the lives of their children. If this is how you feel about your phobia, let me offer this reassurance:

You *can* win freedom from your fears.
You *can* learn to control the distressing mental and physical symptoms of acute anxiety.
You *can* teach yourself to cope with, and in most cases to prevent, panic attacks.

1

And you can do this . . .

Whatever type of phobia you may be suffering from.

No matter how old you are.

Even if you have made unsuccessful attempts to overcome your fears in the past.

Whether you have suffered from a phobia for a few months or for many years.

The purpose of this book is to tell you exactly how to wage war on your phobia and to emerge triumphant. Many thousands have already done so. Now, using the same practical procedures, you too can – *fight your phobia and win!*

What is a phobia?

If you look up the word 'phobia' in a dictionary you will find a definition along these lines: 'A fear, hatred or aversion – especially irrational'. It is distinguished from a state of general, or 'free-floating', anxiety by the fact that there is always some kind of stimulus – a particular situation, activity, animal, person or object – which triggers off the fear.

Incidentally, if your own difficulties are more of the 'free-floating' variety, and you feel mentally and physically tense for no apparent reason, then do read on. The programme described in this book will help you too.

The earliest recorded account of a person suffering from a phobia was written four centuries before the birth of Chirst, by Hippocrates, the father of modern medicine. He described a patient who: ' . . . could not go near a precipice or over a bridge, or beside even the shallowest ditch'. Today we would call such a person an *acrophobic*, which means that he, or she, suffers from a fear of heights.

A more detailed description of phobias was given by the English cleric Robert Burton in his *Anatomy of Melancholy*, published in 1621. Burton wrote of: 'One that durst not walk alone from home for fear he would swoon or die . . . Another dare not go over a bridge, come near a pool, rock, steep hill, lie in a chamber where cross-beams are, for fear that he may be tempted to hang, drown or precipitate himself.'

A phobia, then, is a feeling of fear generated by anything which does not pose a genuine threat to our survival. The response may be mainly a mental one, producing confused thinking, the inability to recall even well-remembered facts and, fairly frequently, a sensation

2

of blind panic. Equally it may be largely a physical reaction, resulting in such handicapping symptoms as a churning stomach, nausea, dizziness, dry mouth, sweating, trembling, blushing, rapidly beating heart, and fast, uneven breathing.

Many phobics, and perhaps you are among them, suffer both mentally and physically, and when this happens these effects tend to feed on each other and, as we shall see, intensify the suffering.

You can become phobic about anything

Although some phobias, for example agoraphobia and claustrophobia, are fairly well known, it is important to understand that one can become phobic about absolutely *anything in the world*. In order to classify such fears, some of the most common have been given specific names, usually created from a Greek word. For example, *agoraphobia* does not, as is widely believed, mean a fear of open spaces. The word is derived from the Greek root *agora* meaning a place of assembly or a market-place. This is a far more accurate reflection of the true source of the agoraphobic's fears for, as I shall explain in the final part of this book, it is *crowded* places, rather than empty beaches or deserted plains, which such people most deeply fear.

Although the list below is far from complete, only a small proportion of phobic responses have ever been given specific names and there was no space to include all of these, it will give you some idea of the astonishingly wide range of fear sources.

Fear of:

Air: aerophobia.
Animals: zoophobia.
Anything new: neophobia; kaino(to)phobia.
Bees: apiphobia.
Being alone: autophobia; monophobia.
Being buried alive: taphephobia.
Being looked at: scopophobia.
Being touched: haphephobia; haptephobia.

Birds: ornithophobia.
Blood: hematophobia.
Blushing: ereuthophobia.
Brain-disease: meningitophobia.
Bridges: gephyrophobia.
Cats: ailurophobia; gatophobia.
· Choking: anginophobia.
Colours: chromatophobia.
Confinement: claustrophobia.
Corpses: necrophobia.

3

Crossing the street:
dromophobia.
Crowds: ochlophobia;
demophobia.
Darkness: scotophobia;
nyctophobia.
Death: thanatophobia.
Depth: bathophobia.
Devil: demonophobia.
Dirt: mysophobia.
Disease: monopathophobia.
Dogs: cynophobia.
Dolls: pediophobia.
Dust: amathophobia.
Eating: phagophobia.
Electricity: electrophobia.
Emptiness: kenophobia.
Excrement: coprophobia.
Feathers: pteronophobia.
Female genitals:
eurotophobia.
Filth: mysophobia:
rupophobia.
Fire: pyrophobia.
Fish: ichthyophobia.
Flying: aviophobia.
Fog: homichlophobia.
Food: cibophobia.
Frogs: batrachophobia.
Ghosts: phasmophobia.
Girls: parthenophobia.
God: theophobia.
Hair: trichopathophobia;
trichophobia.
Height: acrophobia;
hyposophobia.
High objects: batophobia.
House: domatophobia;
oikophobia.
Injury: traumatophobia.
Insects: acarophobia;
entomophobia.

Jealousy: zelophobia.
Knives: aichmophobia.
Lightning: astraphobia;
keraunophobia.
Leaving the house:
agoraphobia.
Machinery: mechanophobia.
Man: androphobia.
Marriage: gamophobia.
Medicine: pharmacophobia.
Money: chrematophobia.
Motion: kinesophobia.
Mice: musophobia.
Naked body: gymnophobia.
Needles: belonephobia.
Night: noctiphobia.
Pain: algophobia;
odynophobia.
Parasites: parasitophobia.
Pleasure: hedonophobia.
Rain: ombrophobia.
Railways:
siderodromophobia.
Red: erythrophobia.
Responsibility:
hypengyophobia.
Rivers: potamophobia.
Sacred things: hierophobia.
Sea: thalassophobia.
Self: autophobia.
Semen: spermatophobia.
Sex: genophobia.
Sexual intercourse:
coitophobia.
Sin: hamartophobia.
Sitting down: kathisophobia.
Skin disease:
dermatosiophobia.
Sleep: hypnophobia.
Snakes: ophidiophobia.
Snow: chionophobia.
Solitude: eremiphobia.

Spiders: arachneophobia.   Travel: hodophobia.
Stairs: climacophobia.   Vehicles: amaxophobia.
Strangers: xenophobia.   Vomit: emetophobia.
Teeth: odontophobia.   Water: hydrophobia.
Thirteen: triskaidekaphobia.   Wind: anemophobia.
Thunder: brontophobia;   Women: gynophobia.
  astrophobia.   Writing: graphophobia.

Fear and avoidance

From that list you can see that while some of the items could not, realistically, be regarded as in any way hazardous others could pose a potential threat to life and limb. For instance, this would be true of disease, electricity, lightning, machinery, spiders and snakes. There are others which, although generally safe, do contain a slight element of risk, such as aircraft, bridges, dogs, thunder, trains, wind, and water. Finally there are things which, while not threatening to life and limb, are regarded as so unpleasant that most people, whether phobic or not, prefer not to have any contact with them. For example, blood, vomit, excrement and corpses.

All these, as well as many other objects and animals, situations and circumstances, places, people, and activities arouse justifiable feelings of apprehension and a desire to avoid them. So at what point does a reasonable amount of anxiety and avoidance become a phobia?

Where apparently safe items are concerned, it is fair to say that *any* anxiety indicates a phobic response. For example, somebody who feels fear at the sight of a small spider, a kitten, human hair, or earthworm probably does not have a phobia about them.

When some risk is involved, then whether or not a phobia is present depends on whether the amount of anxiety bears any relation to the degree of danger involved. Many people feel slightly apprehensive when they board a jet aircraft, especially if they are not used to flying. But to be so stricken by panic that one always avoids air travel, or can only undertake it after taking tranquillizers (or liberal amounts of alcohol) indicates a phobic response.

Some people with mild phobias manage reasonably well, simply by avoiding those things which make them afraid. Whether or not this tactic is successful depends on the type and intensity of the phobic response. Somebody slightly fearful of spiders, for instance, might cope by killing any which come in range with a rolled-up newspaper and washing down the drain any spider unfortunate enough to emerge in their bath.

While this may be bad news for spiders it does allow the mildly spider phobic man or woman to live with their fears. But if spiders produced much greater anxiety this strategy would probably fail. Because the sufferer panics at the sight of even a small spider the avoidance is all the greater. For example he, or she, might not even enter the bathroom until their partner had checked the bath. If living alone, the phobic might be fearful even to enter any room where a spider had been seen.

The greater the anxiety, the stronger is the desire to avoid what is feared. But, at the same time, the greater the avoidance the more disruption will be caused to that person's way of life. The best way to illustrate this is to let an insect phobic describe her own response to these fears:

> From about the end of May onwards I hardly ever leave the house. Even on the hottest day I stay indoors, usually in my bedroom which I have made virtually insect proof. I place sticky tape around all the windows and seal the doors as best I can. I have put insect screens up. The house often gets like an oven in the summer. My husband and two children have to go on holiday without me, and this makes me very, very unhappy. I can't watch television, even programmes which have nothing to do with natural history some-times show pictures of insects and I dare not take the risk. My husband goes through magazines and newspapers before I read them and takes out all mention of insects. I spray the house dozens of times a day from May to late November But even during the winter, when I do feel less anxious, I can never sleep away from home – not even in a friend's house. The thought of an insect, especially flying ones, makes me feel physically ill. My nerves get in a dreadful state and I have terrible headaches.

Sometimes phobias which might not, at first sight, appear to be particularly disruptive, turn out to be terribly restricting. A person unable to pass over or under any kind of bridge could be confined to travelling within a very limited area around his, or her, home. Think for a moment how far you could walk or drive without encountering a bridge.

Similarly, a phobic reaction to something most people merely regard as unpleasant can have unexpectedly far-reaching consequences. A needle phobic will avoid going to the dentist, refuse to have the shots needed for travel to many parts of the world, be fearful of having even a minor operation. A blood phobic might be unable to care for his, or her, children if they cut or graze themselves. Even more restricting can be the reactions of a vomit phobic, as this account by a twenty-three-year-old girl sufferer reveals:

> Since my fear first developed my social life has almost disappeared. I am unable to go out at all on Saturday night because I am sure I will see a drunk being ill. I haven't had a holiday for three years because I dare not fly or go on a boat. I avoid trains as well. I had to change my job, which I really enjoyed, because I couldn't face the bus ride to the office. My new job is boring, but I can walk all the way. I used to like eating out, but now I am afraid somebody might be ill in the restaurant or I might eat something which disagreed with me. I no longer have a boyfriend as I am terrified of getting pregnant and suffering morning sickness. I used to enjoy curries and spicy dishes, but now I only eat very bland, unsalted food in case it makes me ill. When I get a headache or have flu I can't take a tablet because it might make me ill.

'They that live in fear,' wrote Robert Burton, 'are never free, resolute, secure, merry, but in continual pain . . . No greater misery, no rack, no torture like unto it.' Three centuries later such fear still rules the lives of a multitude of people suffering from phobias.

2

What Not to Believe About Your Phobia

As if having a phobia was not painful enough many phobia sufferers and their well-meaning families or friends make matters worse by holding one or more seriously mistaken views about the nature of phobias and anxiety, and the ways in which such fears can best be removed. Before starting to fight your phobia it is essential to understand the truth about these fears and to rid yourself of the following misconceptions:

'I must be going mad . . .'

Because phobias appear so irrational, and the symptoms are so distressing, many people suffering from them come to the conclusion that their fears are a sign of insanity. This is probably the most damaging of the false beliefs because, by increasing general anxiety, it can easily intensify the phobia itself. As mental and physical symptoms grow stronger so too does the sufferer's conviction that he, or she, must be taking leave of their senses. On occasions this 'fear of the fear' can transform a relatively mild and initially limited phobia into a more powerful and restricting reaction.

Suppose, for example, a woman develops a phobia about cats. In the past, she was very fond of them. But soon even the sight of a small, fluffy, kitten arouses anxiety. If she comes across one accidentally she feels sick and faint, her heart begins to race, and her legs tremble. Sometimes the panic is so acute she flees from the room. She thinks: 'Only somebody who was a little crazy could ever feel *that* frightened of cats . . . I must be off my head!'

Not surprisingly such thoughts make her even more anxious, and mean that any encounter with cats – even seeing them on television or looking at pictures of them in a book – will produce intense fear. These feelings, in turn, support her belief that she is mentally unbalanced, and so increase the anxiety still further. In time her difficulties may reach the point where professional help from a psychologist or a psychiatrist becomes necessary. But it was her worry over the *nature* of the phobia, completely unfounded, rather than the phobia itself, which had led to this state of affairs.

So let me make the point absolutely clear: *A phobia is not a serious mental illness (such as schizophrenia) nor is it connected with any known physical illness.*

However painful and distressing your symptoms, no matter how irrational and inexplicable your phobia and its effects may seem, no matter how dramatic and complete your loss of mental and/or physical control, you must not see in your phobia the first signs of insanity. Neither does it indicate that you are on the verge of a 'nervous breakdown'.

The modern view of phobias, which is accepted by the majority of specialists and supported by a wealth of clinical and research evidence, is that they come about as the result of an unfortunate but entirely normal process of learning. This is a crucial point to which I will be returning later on.

'*A phobia is a very rare and little-understood problem . . .*'

Largely because of the secrecy which surrounds the disability, many phobics believe themselves to be suffering from an unusual complaint. The fact that their fears are aroused by things which are being coped with effortlessly by everyone else they know, will support this view. 'Surely', they think, 'I must be the victim of a rare and unique illness about which little is known and nothing can be done.' This too is an entirely mistaken notion.

Phobias are, in fact, extremely common. Although nobody knows exactly how many suffer from a phobia serious enough to disrupt their lives significantly, studies suggest that as many as one person in ten experiences such difficulties at least once in their life. Given that this estimate is accurate, and most experts agree it is a reasonable one, then Britain, Europe, Scandinavia, the United States and Canada have, between them, some fifty-five million people with seriously disruptive phobias. Far from being uncommon, your phobia simply qualifies you for membership of the world's least exclusive club!

As for there not being any real understanding of the problem, or any effective means of treatment, this too is completely false. Phobias have been studied by psychologists, psychiatrists and doctors for well over a hundred years and, although much more certainly remains to be discovered and understood, a great deal is now known about them. Over the past thirty years increasingly effective treatment procedures have been developed, mostly using clinical and research findings from the field of behavioural psychology. Today a vast body of knowledge about all types of phobia exists, and sufferers can be treated with considerable success.

The trouble is that the first person a phobia sufferer usually sees is the family doctor and he, or she, may not always be the best person to give help and advice. There are two reasons for this. The first is that phobias are most effectively treated using psychological rather than medical procedures.

In the past, while doctors were well trained in medicine they were not usually given much training in psychology. Although the situation has greatly improved in recent years, the first response of many GPs on learning that a patient has phobic difficulties is to reach for the pad and write out a prescription for some type of tranquillizer, most often Valium or Librium.

In fairness to doctors two points must be made. The first is that they are very short of time, and advising patients how best to overcome their phobias using psychological procedures is a lengthy business. It must also be said that many patients expect to be given a pill or a potion when they visit their GP and feel rather cheated if they have to leave the consulting room empty handed.

Unfortunately, while tranquillizers can ease the symptoms of anxiety in the short-term, the role in which they are most beneficial, they do not offer any long-term answers. Often the best answer is to obtain the benefits such drugs provide *while* you master the skills needed to combat your anxiety in the long-term by using the body's natural powers.

If you are currently taking tranquillizers then you *must* continue to do so when working through this programme. As you learn natural procedures for controlling anxiety it may well be possible, gradually, to reduce your dependency on drugs. But such changes should only be made on the advice of your doctor.

'*I must be weak-willed or very stupid to have a phobia. . .*'

Phobics often consider themselves 'stupid' or 'weak', because that's what other people are constantly telling them. Because the fear seems so irrational, non-sufferers frequently react with impatience and irritation when the phobic is unable to do something which most people tackle with ease.

'I don't care much for spiders', the wife of a thirty-two-year-old salesman told me, 'but John just loses all control. He runs out of the room. If he tries to stay he goes pale and starts to tremble. He says he will faint or be sick. It's so stupid and unmanly.'

Such charges are entirely false. Phobias are nothing to do with age, education, intellect or income. They are not due to a fault in your character or a flaw in your personality. They are certainly not an indication of weakness. Indeed, some of the bravest people I know are phobics fighting to free themselves of their fears. So, if non-phobics ever deride you for being 'foolish', or exhort you to 'face up to your fears' and to 'pull yourself together', if they dismiss your anxiety as 'absurd' and accuse you of defects in personality or character, do not allow your self-esteem to wither and your self-confidence to wilt under their verbal assaults.

They speak with the voice of ignorance about fears they simply do not understand. But then, only somebody who has suffered, or is suffering, the distress produced by a phobia can truly appreciate your own anxiety.

'Positive thinking will cure your phobia . . .'

While positive thinking is an important part of any treatment prog-ramme, it must be the right kind of positive thinking. Telling yourself – or being told – to exercise 'self-control', and expecting that this will get rid of the fears, is as futile as believing you can swim without lessons, merely by an effort of will. Plunge into the deep-end in either case and you are going to find yourself right out of your depth.

'I am not going to feel afraid when I board that aircraft', an air travel phobic assures himself. But once aboard the jet he feels terrified. Positive thinking having failed, he regards his fears as being beyond control.

'I will stay cool, calm and collected in the supermarket' says the agoraphobic. But she suffers a panic attack all the same and is plunged into despair.

In the training programme, I am going to explain exactly how to use positive thinking in a constructive way so that it makes dealing with phobias easier and leads to success, rather than loss of pride and failure of self-confidence. But remember, unrealistic positive think-ing is going to hinder rather than help you, while will-power alone can never get rid of your phobia. If it could there would be far fewer phobics, because all those I have met desperately wanted to bid their phobia goodbye.

Any phobia is unpleasant. Some are so restricting that they shackle the victim to a lifestyle that is both deeply depressing and very frustrating – a way of living which offers little stimulation or pleasure and seems to lead only to an equally unattractive tomorrow. How does such a difficulty arise? Why should otherwise clever, competent, healthy and sensible individuals suffer from something so seemingly irrational?

I have stressed that a phobia is *not* a form of serious mental illness. Nor is it something you are born with. And it does *not* arise because you have a defect in personality or a weakness of character. A phobia is certainly nothing to feel ashamed about. Neither is it a burden which can be set down through effort of will alone.

To understand how and why phobias occur we will have to look at the idea of *learning* in what may strike you as a novel and rather unexpected way.

3

How You Learn to be Phobic

Infants, as parents well know, are fearless explorers. For them the world is a place of endless fascination to be investigated boldly, to be touched, held, squeezed and – whenever possible – tasted! Crawling or toddling eagerly towards the next great adventure, they are interested in almost everything and afraid of hardly anything.

Before very long, however, their innocent enthusiasm is tempered by caution. They rapidly realize that there are painful as well as pleasurable discoveries to be made. They find out that certain things bring hurt instead of happiness and that satisfying one's curiosity can be a frightening affair.

Sometimes they discover this by direct experience. The warm and fluffy object they joyously cuddle turns out to be a very unfriendly cat. That pretty yellow paste which looked so appetizing in the jar on the kitchen shelf is actually a very nasty thing called mustard. The tin can which looked such an attractive toy has a serrated edge which draws blood – and fear-stricken tears.

More often, however, the fears of adults teach children to become afraid. They learn from Mother's warning cry as they reach for the saucepan of boiling water, from Father's shout of horror as he snatches them from the sill of a carelessly-opened first floor window, and from all the scoldings and punishments intended to stop them from doing or saying anything of which adults disapprove.

If they are to survive – physically and socially – children must be taught to avoid those activities and objects, animals, people and places that could do them harm. In order to learn avoidance the child must first learn to feel afraid.

Learning to fear

In 1920, a psychologist named John Broadus Watson carried out an experiment which provided a classic illustration of how children – and adults – learn to fear. His subject, who has gone down in scientific history by the name of Little Albert, was an eleven-month-old orphan who was fond of white rats. After observing the child for some while and noting the fearless way in which he approached and handled the animals, Watson stood behind the child with a hammer and a sheet of metal. Each time Little Albert reached out to touch a rat, Watson struck hammer and metal together with an earsplitting crash. Naturally the deafening noise startled and scared Little Albert.

After a while, because the frightening sounds became linked to the sight of the rats, Little Albert was no longer willing to touch or play with the animals. Indeed, even the sight of them made him cry and try to escape. To use a piece of jargon, Little Albert had been *conditioned* to fear white rats. In other words he was now *phobic* about them. You will be relieved to know that, having demonstrated his theory about how phobias arise, Watson set about eliminating the boy's fears by using procedures similar to those which I shall be describing in the training programme.

Phobias and fears

From what I have said so far, two points will – I hope – have become clear to you. The first is that anxiety is not only a perfectly natural and normal response, but one which is essential to our survival. It ensures that we learn to avoid, or to be very careful when dealing with, anything in life which is hazardous or harmful. The greater we perceive the threat to be, the greater the anxiety aroused and the stronger our desire for escape or avoidance. An equally vital effect of anxiety, and one which I will look at in more detail later, is to 'tune up' mind and body so that we can handle the feared situation with the best possible chance of success.

Secondly we come to attach the label 'fear this' and 'avoid that' to certain things, as a result of learning. We are not born with the notion that any particular object is dangerous or threatening. Having said that, I must add that research has shown that we do possess an inborn tendency to fear certain kinds of things more than others. Infants are more likely to become afraid of things which move, for example, than those which remain motionless.

Psychologists who attempted to condition infants to fear objects like a building-block or a hairbrush, using Watson's technique, were unable to do so. This fact led Sigmund Freud, the founder of psychoanalysis, to distinguish two kinds of phobic responses according to the nature of the feared object. There were 'common phobias', which he saw as an exaggerated fear of all those things which everybody detests or fears to some extent, such as night, solitude, death, illness, dangers in general, snakes etc., and 'specific phobias', the fear of special circumstances that inspire no fear in the normal man.

So far as the treatment of phobias is concerned, however, it makes no difference whether the response is an intense reaction to things which make most people slightly fearful or acute anxiety generated by objects others see no cause to fear. Exactly the same procedures may be employed to eliminate them from your life.

As you will now understand, your phobia is really a conditioned response producing anxiety. For various reasons – and I will explore these in more detail – you have learned to attach the 'fears' label to something most people either do not fear at all or only to a minor and non-disruptive extent. But the processes by which this has occurred – anxiety arousal and learning – are both perfectly normal.

Rewards which make learning more rapid

A very important concept in psychology, one which has been around since the late nineteenth century, is called the *Law of Effect*. This states that when you do something which has a positive result the chances are that you will repeat that action. If what you do has negative consequences, however, you will be less likely to do it.

In everyday terms, if Johnny does the washing-up and Mary mows the lawn without being asked or told to do so, then whether or not they repeat those helpful deeds depends on how their parents respond. Immediate praise will increase the likelihood while critical comments about the way those tasks were carried out decreases that probability.

This may sound more like a matter of simple common sense than a particular psychological law. But in fact, the relationship between behaviour and rewards is a good deal more complex and subtle than those examples suggest. Suppose, for example, Johnny's parents wait a week before giving him a hefty increase in pocket-money as a token of their pleasure. Will this be more, or less, effective than immediate praise? How will Mary respond if her parents offer her praise on some occasions when she helps in the garden, but ignore her efforts at other times?

Contrary to what many people might think, research has shown that the critical factor is usually the amount of time which passes between doing something and receiving a reward rather than the size of that reward. The shorter the delay the more effective that reward will be in encouraging somebody to act in a particular way. The longer the delay the less powerful its influence.

Furthermore, occasional rewards, handed out on a random basis, will build a pattern of behaviour more quickly and strongly than if they are provided consistently. One can observe the power of rewards which are distributed randomly but when they do occur are provided immediately, by looking at the behaviour of people gambling with fruit-machines. These aptly-named one-armed bandits make their payments in an apparently haphazard manner. Nobody can say how many pulls on the handle, or how much time, will pass between one pay-out and the next. But when the reward does come it is virtually instantaneous. The tumblers click up a winning sequence and the gambler is greeted by the joyous sound of coins cascading into the tray.

Do the winnings go into the gambler's pocket and stay there as he, or she, walks quickly away from the bandit? Of course not. Psychology is on the side of those who own the fruit-machines. Most punters keep right on playing, and almost always end up losing their short-lived gains. Immediate rewards, made randomly, have conditioned the players to a very special piece of behaviour – pulling the lever and watching the tumblers spin. They have certainly not trained the gambler to take the money and run!

What has all this got to do with your phobia? The answer is, a very great deal. You too have acquired a phobic response through the same combination of immediate rewards randomly applied.

When NOT doing something brings rewards

So far we have only looked at rewards in positive terms as things which are pleasing and desirable. This type of consequence is known, in technical terms, as a 'positive reinforcement'. But there are also so-called 'negative reinforcements', which act as equally powerful rewards. A negative reinforcer occurs any time we escape from, or avoid, an unpleasant and distressing situation.

If you are performing a task which makes you anxious, then anything which stops you from carrying on with it will be negatively reinforced. In other words the removal of that anxiety will provide an immediate, and powerful, reward. Here's how it might work in real life.

A husband and wife have been arguing because she wants to take a job outside the home while he wants her to remain a housewife. The row makes the wife very anxious. In order to bring their discussion to a halt she agrees not to look for employment.

The husband has been *positively reinforced* for his refusal to allow his wife to go out to work while she has been *negatively reinforced* (through the removal of anxiety) for giving in to him. If they quarrel in the future it is now slightly more probable that he will insist on getting his own way while she will give in to him.

This interplay of positive and negative reinforcement is often an important factor in creating patterns of behaviour between a phobic and his, or her, partner. For instance, in agoraphobia, the wife may ask her husband to undertake all the tasks which make her fearful, such as doing the shopping, picking up the children from school, and so on. His agreement, although kindly meant, actually strengthens her desire to stay at home (through negative reinforcement and the reduction of anxiety). At the same time her pleasure and relief, which any loving partner will welcome, positively reinforces his willingness to take those burdens off her hands. Although the help was given out of the best possible motives, the likely result of this exchange of rewards is that her agoraphobia will become ever more firmly entrenched.

Incidently, if you are currently helping an agoraphobic in this way, I am certainly not suggesting that you should abruptly withdraw your assistance. Such a response would be both inappropriate and very unhelpful. Later in the book I will explain exactly how the family and friends of an agoraphobic can provide the right sort of help, advice and encouragement.

4

SAAR – The Phobia Builder

The way in which phobias arise is well illustrated by the case history of Caroline.

We first met when she was forty-six years old and had been a dog phobic for four years. At that time her phobia was having an extremely damaging effect on her marriage and social life. She was unwilling to leave home, except by car, and could not go shopping. She was too frightened to board trains or buses and never dared go out into the country, although previously she had adored going for long walks over the hills. Now the risk of encountering a dog was too great. She refused to see friends who owned dogs and could only look at television programmes when certain that no dogs would be featured. The sight of a puppy in the street was enough to provoke a panic attack. Even discussing her fears with a therapist aroused considerable anxiety.

Here is how she described the way those fears arose . . .

I went to see my married sister and she had a neighbour over for coffee. This woman had a large dog, I forget the breed but it may have been an Alsatian. It was lying right across the door and I had to step over it. Soon after I sat down it came and sat beside me. I felt nervous, although up to that time I had not been the least bit worried by dogs . . . it was a small room and the seats were quite low. The dog seemed to be watching me. His mouth was open and I could see saliva dribbling from his tongue . . . his owner did nothing to call him back. I became increasingly anxious and flustered. The dog suddenly lunged, not hard and only in play, but he sent my cup flying. I had to go out of the room to wash and sponge my dress. The owner was very apologetic, but when I came back into the room she had not removed her dog. I began to be very nervous indeed. I felt hot and rather sick. In the end I couldn't stand it any longer.

I made an excuse to my sister and went home. A few days later – I had almost forgotten the first incident – I saw a dogfight in the street. I felt very tense and crossed over the road to avoid them. From then on I always made a point of walking on the other side of the street if I saw a big dog, even if it was on a leash. After a time much smaller dogs made me feel anxious . . . One day a friend called on me with a miniature poodle, it was a pint-sized creature but I felt as nervous with it in the room as I had with the Alsatian . . .

Caroline's story shows how just two frightening encounters with dogs were sufficient to sow the seeds from which her phobia grew. The animals were the trigger, or stimulus (S) which produced consider- able anxiety (A) and a strong need for avoidance (A) which led to her fears subsiding. This provided Caroline with a reward (R) for her response. An analysis of the process reveals the following pattern:

Stimulus . . . Anxiety . . . Avoidance . . . Reward.

(S)   **(A)**   **(A)**   **(R)**

All types of phobic reaction develop as a result of the same sequence of events. SAAR, therefore, makes up the set of psychological building blocks from which a phobia is created.

S – *Stimulus*
Whatever it is that makes you feel anxious or afraid. While your phobia is developing this could be something you have to see or do, somewhere you have to go, or people you must meet. Later, with the phobic reaction entrenched, merely thinking about the feared stimulus way prove sufficient to produce a high level of . . .

A – *Anxiety*
The mental and physical symptoms of a high level of anxiety are painful, and disruptive in themselves. No matter what you are attempting to do, intense anxiety ensures you will do it worse. To get rid of these feelings you are likely to attempt some form of . . .

A – *Avoidance*
When merely thinking about the fear stimulus makes you afraid, the avoidance may be mental. This does not mean, however, that you drive all thoughts of it from your mind. Indeed some phobics constantly dwell on their anxieties and can think of very little else. But their ideas are almost always negative and couched in terms of *not* being able to cope.

They see themselves trying to overcome their phobia and failing miserably, of losing control and becoming the centre of critical attention and of having a panic attack and being made to look foolish. The avoidance comes in never seeing themselves confronting and coping with the feared situation.

When the possibility of having to face their fears in real life arises, the immediate response is often the conviction that the challenge is beyond them and excuses for not doing it must be found. In real life, the avoidance may take a more obvious form, with the phobic doing or saying almost anything in order to get away from the stimulus. As we have seen, such avoidance brings a rapid . . .

R – *Reward*
The more powerful the original anxiety and the more successful the avoidance, the stronger this reward will prove, as the mental and physical anxiety symptoms disappear. The greater the reward the more likely it is you will try and avoid the fear stimulus in future. The more intense the subsequent anxiety is, the more probable avoidance becomes.

Now let's look at two more case histories which show this process in action.

Susan — a railway platform phobic Susan's phobia about underground platforms developed much more rapidly than Caroline's fear of dogs. Indeed her transformation from a regular and untroubled traveller to a phobic occurred in the few seconds it took to experience a severe panic attack.

My problems started one evening about twenty years ago. I was standing near the edge of a station platform waiting for my usual train home. I had been travelling to and from this particular station for some twenty-five years. I was reading an evening paper and, as I turned over a page, I glimpsed the live rail. What happened in that split second I'll never know. I was suddenly petrified but rooted to the spot. Then I had to rush out. I couldn't bring myself to go back onto the platform. In the end I travelled home by bus. Now I cannot go anywhere by train.

I was forced to leave my job, which I enjoyed, and find work closer to home so that I didn't have to commute by train. As trains are much the most convenient form of transport, not being able to use them is very restricting. If I want to travel into town to have a meal, see friends or go to the films I usually have to come home by taxi and the extra expense makes it impossible for me to afford many outings.

Here again we see the powerful SAAR at work building Susan's phobia from the original panic attack, by means of avoidance and reward.

Mark — a social phobic At the time Mark's phobia of other people began he was aged twenty-three and living in a small religious community. His intention was to become a priest.

I can remember very clearly when my difficulties first began. I had been feeling rather depressed for several months and was being treated by my doctor. One morning I went down to the dining room for lunch and started to eat. I usually sat opposite a friend but today he was away and I found myself confronted by a stranger.

I was suddenly overwhelmed by a blinding panic. I knew that I had to get out of the room or I would faint or something. My heart was racing and my whole body trembled. I rushed to my bedroom. That evening I said I felt ill and avoided going down for dinner. The following morning hunger drove me down to the dining room but I immediately felt terribly anxious. From then on it became impossible for me to eat in the dining room. The other people were very sympathetic and let me take my meals in the kitchen.

I could only eat in a room which had less than four people in it. Gradually it was not just a question of eating in semi-private. I couldn't even be in a room with other people. I cut myself off from all my friends. I felt that, if I went outside, everybody was looking at me . . .

My whole life changed. I didn't seem to be able to control anything about the way I felt. If I went into a room and found somebody else there I would get the feeling: 'I've got to get out of here.' I tried to tell myself: 'Sit down . . . stop acting crazy.' But it was no good – I just had to get up and go!

Here we can see how the original panic attack in the presence of an unexpected stranger led to rapid avoidance and a correspondingly powerful reward as the fear subsided. Mark's account also shows the way in which a fairly specific stimulus – in his case eating in the community dining hall – can rapidly extend to cover a large number of similar situations. Mark was obliged to leave the community and spent several miserable years a virtual prisoner in his parents' home, before he found the help needed to overcome his fears. Today, fully recovered, he is a teacher.

How phobias are sustained

You may perhaps be wondering why, after a long period of avoidance, the phobia does not simply disappear. Surely by more or less permanently removing the anxiety source the phobic takes away the reward which, as I have explained, sustains the fear. The answer lies in the potency of occasional rewards.

Think back to our fruit-machine addict, patiently pulling the handle and putting in his money. Although he loses far more frequently than he wins, those few times that he does hit the jack-pot are sufficient to sustain his strong desire to play on fruit-machines.

Phobias are maintained by a similar process. It only takes occasional avoidance, resulting in a reduction in anxiety, to preserve the fear response. Nor does this avoidance have to occur in real life. It is quite sufficient if it only happens in the imagination.

Here's how it could work for Caroline . . . 'Let's go for a walk in the country on Saturday', her husband suggests in the middle of the week. Caroline hesitantly agrees. As the weekend approaches, she feels increasingly afraid. In her mind's eye she pictures terrifying encounters with a whole kennel load of snarling, snapping, savage dogs. On Saturday morning she complains of a bad headache as an excuse not to have to go out.

The fear stimulus only appeared in her imagination, but the anxiety and the avoidance were all too real. If Caroline only responds in that way once every few weeks the reward will still prove sufficient to sustain her phobia at a high level.

Some people are at more risk than others

Many people have frightening encounters with animals, endure moments of blind panic in certain situations or become extremely anxious when carrying out some activity, yet never develop a phobia. So why do incidents which leave most of us relatively unscathed lead to phobias in others? As yet, there is no certain answer to this important question.

If we knew exactly why some individuals are more at risk than others it might be possible to safeguard them in some way. However, all the research indicates that two factors are likely to be involved.

Firstly, some people appear to be more vulnerable to phobias because of the way their nervous systems function. Secondly, the chances of becoming phobic increase when a person is stressed by physical ill-health or serious emotional problems.

Phobias and your personality

You have only to think about some of your friends and acquaintances to appreciate how very differently individuals respond to life. Some are lively, voluble, open, and sociable. They are good at forming relationships, enjoy the company of others and are eager to take up fresh challenges. Others are quieter and more self-sufficient. They may find it more difficult to be very sociable and so have fewer friends. Many years ago the Swiss psychologist Carl Jung named these distinct personality types *extravert* and *introvert*.

Today psychologists attribute such differences in outlook and behaviour to the differing amounts of stimulation which an individual's nervous system requires in order to function effectively. Extraverts, it is thought, require a considerable amount of regular stimulation to stay healthy and happy. Introverts, on the other hand, have a far lower need for stimulation.

One result is that introverts tend to learn faster than extraverts. Sometimes just one experience is sufficient to teach them a permanent lesson. If an introverted child is punished for being naughty, he or she is much less likely to offend again than the extravert youngster who might be punished on numerous occasions without mending his or her ways.

The significance of this in terms of phobias is obvious. We would expect introverts, with their ability to learn more rapidly, to become phobic more often than extraverts. This in fact is what studies of the personality of phobics have revealed. You should not come to the conclusion, however, that if you happen to be rather more of an introvert than an extravert you will inevitably develop a phobia. The vast majority of introverts never suffer in this way. All one can say is that introverted men and women may be at slightly greater risk than extraverts.

Phobias and life events

Everybody, even reasonably extraverted individuals, becomes more vulnerable if suffering from poor health or while passing through a major emotional upheaval. Psychologists have termed such periods of crisis – *Life-Events*. These include . . .*

1 Bereavement.
2 The loss of one's job – especially through redundancy.
3 Sickness in the family.
4 Financial difficulties.
5 Divorce or the loss of an intimate relationship.
6 Moving to a strange neighbourhood.
7 Women seem to be more at risk during the days immediately prior

to menstruation and after childbirth, especially if there were any complications.

The greater the number of life events you are trying to cope with, especially if the emotional crisis comes at a time when you are physically run-down, the more vulnerable you are likely to be. But if you are currently going through a difficult time, please do not read more into this statement than is actually there.

Mental stress and/or physical ill-health do not inevitably mean you will become a phobic. Indeed, all the evidence shows that most people are able to survive extremely stressful life events without ever developing a phobia.

5

The 'Fight or Flight' Response

Whenever you grow anxious a number of unpleasant things start happening. The first sign that all is not well is often felt as a rather sickening lurch in the pit of your stomach. This will usually be followed by some, or all, of the following: an increase in heart rate, rapid and irregular breathing, a dry mouth and a feeling that you are going to be sick. Your head feels either very light or very heavy, sometimes both in rapid succession. You are giddy and begin to tremble. You may blush, or go very white. You fear you are going to faint. You may perspire profusely, yet somehow manage to feel shivery at the same time.

Your mind becomes confused. Rational thoughts and sensible ideas take flight leaving you prey to a host of wild and usually extremely negative thoughts: 'I can't cope . . . I am going to lose control . . . I must get away . . .'. During initial anxiety attacks many sufferers are convinced they are about to have a heart attack and die. When the fear finally passes you are left weak, wretched and depressed.

The experience of acute anxiety is very, very unpleasant. But why does it happen at all? How is it that the human body is capable of something so seemingly painful and apparently unhelpful as the anxiety response?

The same could, of course, be said about pain. Yet, as most people realize, this has a very important role to play in our survival. Its purpose is to warn us that something is going wrong with the system so that we can take steps to put matters right before lasting damage is done. There are, in fact, some people who are incapable of feeling pain. Far from being blessed with a wonderful freedom from discomfort these unfortunate individuals are actually cursed with a dreadful disability. They can cut, burn, bruise, and scald themselves terribly, only realizing how much harm has been done when they see the extent of their injuries.

Anxiety, like pain, is there to ensure survival. It alerts us to danger and motivates us to escape from, or to avoid, life-threatening situations.

Imagine one of our early ancestors on a search for food in hostile terrain. Suddenly he hears a sound from the nearby undergrowth. His body must respond instantly to the possibility of an attack by man or beast. If danger really threatens, the hunter will have to do one of two things – stand and fight, or turn and flee. In order to do either successfully crucial changes will have to take place in the way his body is functioning.

How anxiety alters your body

To fight or to flee effectively, arm and leg muscles must be given more food (glycogen) and oxygen in order to increase their strength and stamina. Strenuous activity produces additional amounts of waste products, such as carbon dioxide, which must be transported away from the cells and expelled from the body as quickly as possible.

Increased heart rate pushes the blood around the system more rapidly, carrying in the urgently-needed oxygen and removing the unwanted by-products. Rapid breathing speeds up the rate at which oxygen is taken into the body and carbon dioxide is pushed out.

There are other, less obvious, changes as well. The liver releases extra supplies of glycocen. The blood chemistry is subtly altered so that it will clot more swiftly should an injury occur.

It is rather like a battle cruiser steaming into action. As the alert klaxon sounds, sailors are taken from such temporarily non-essential departments as the laundry, galley and bakery in order to man guns. In the human body some departments are also 'closed down' for the duration of the emergency so that every ounce of strength and energy can be expended on the urgent business of ensuring survival.

Digestion is slowed, blood is diverted from the stomach and skin and sent in greater quantities to the muscles of the arms and legs and to the brain. The result is a dry mouth, upset stomach and pale skin. To get rid of the extra heat produced by increased activity we start to perspire. If the body temperature drops too sharply, however, steps are immediately taken to trap the heat.

Animals achieve this by raising their body hairs. We do it too, but having less body hair the result is usually goose-pimples as the skin attempts to erect its non-existent hairs. The expression 'being so frightened your hair stands on end' does, therefore, have a foundation in biological truth. For our primitive hunter this virtually instantaneous response might well have meant the difference between life and death.

Survival in the modern jungle

Even today, there are times when the anxiety response is still a life-saver. Newspaper stories often recount how, at moments of extreme danger, ordinary men and women have found themselves capable of feats demanding great agility, tremendous strength, fleetness of foot and enormous endurance.

A mother lifts a fallen tree from her crushed car to pull her child to safety. A frail elderly person fights off an assault by a muscled young attacker. A father swims through mountainous seas to save his son from drowning. In each case, those reserves of power could only be called on thanks to the intense physical reaction of the anxiety response.

The trouble is, of course, that survival in the twentieth-century jungle very seldom involves either fight or flight in the literal sense. Typically we have to deal with dangers that put at risk not our physical survival but our emotional or intellectual well-being. For example, many people grow extremely anxious when . . .

1 Faced by verbal aggression despite the fact there is no risk of physical violence.
2 Rejected by somebody they love, even though a broken heart shows no trace of physical injury.
3 Attempting a task they believe is beyond them, although only their pride will be wounded by failure.
4 Confronted by any situations, objects, people, places, activities or animals which, through the process of learning described in the last chapter, they regard as threatening.

As anxiety increases so too may the conviction that all control has been lost. But that is not entirely correct. Control has not so much been lost as passed to a different part of the brain.

When the Automatic Pilot takes over

We seldom have any choice whether or not to feel afraid. A sudden noise, an unexpected movement, the realization that something terrible is about to happen, trigger off what is called the *startle response*. This is the response that makes you jump when a car backfires, when you hear a sudden movement in the bushes while walking alone through a park at dusk, or when you are driving a car which skids on ice.

Instantly you switch from a fairly relaxed state into one of high 'arousal'. Often, only after the danger has passed, are you aware of the physical effects of the startle response. Such instant switching, without the need, or indeed the possibility, of voluntary control is achieved because our nervous system consists of two parts.

There is the central nervous system, the communications network by which the brain sends its commands to different parts of the body and so controls such voluntary actions as turning over the pages of this book.

But, as you are reading these words, a great many vital bodily functions are taking place without your having to give them the slightest thought. Your heart is beating at a rate of about seventy-two times a minute in order to pump blood around the body. You are breathing rhythmically. Any recently-eaten food is being digested. Your core temperature is being maintained at 98.4°Fahrenheit. All these, and many other extremely complex activities essential to life, are being directed and co-ordinated by far older and much more primitive portions of the brain. Messages from these centres deep within the skull speed to all parts of the body via a specialized communications network called the Autonomic Nervous System (ANS).

We can compare the ANS to the automatic pilot in a modern aircraft. Having switched on their autopilot, the crew can sit back and relax. Thanks to our ANS automatic pilot we are able to live our lives without having to give constant thought to routine bodily functions. By 'flying' our body in this way, the ANS allows us to think, to plan, to solve problems, and to dream dreams. Just imagine trying to do any of those things if you had to tell your heart to keep beating, your lungs to keep filling and emptying, your kidneys to keep producing urine and your stomach to continue digesting lunch!

The problem is, that because the automatic pilot operates largely independently from what we might term the 'thinking brain', it is not normally possible to give it instructions. You cannot, by an effort of will, order your heart to stop beating or your stomach to cease digestion. You cannot, for any length of time, stop breathing. Hold your breath for more than a few minutes and the automatic pilot simply snatches back control and forces you to gasp for air.

It used to be believed that the central nervous system could exert no control at all over the ANS. We now know that this is not entirely so. After special training it is possible to manipulate the ANS to a remarkable extent. Eastern Yogis have long been aware of this, of course, and can slow their heart rates and lower their blood pressure at will. It is only recently, however, that such an ability has been demonstrated to the satisfaction of scientists. Recent experiments using biofeedback equipment – electronic machines which monitor various bodily systems – have shown that almost anybody can learn to do much the same. But, without lengthy and special training, such control is not possible.

In practice this means that when the automatic pilot orders emergency running the 'thinking brain' can do absolutely nothing to countermand that command. You may know, perfectly well, that there is no threat to your survival. It makes no difference. Your automatic pilot believes it poses a threat and responds accordingly. All you can do is experience the consequences.

Speed-up, slow-down

So far I have talked about the *fight or flight* mechanism as if it was a single system. In fact it consists of two branches which work together, most of the time, to produce a normal state of arousal.

They are sometimes compared to the reins of a horse. As every rider knows, equal pressure is used to keep a horse moving in a straight line. When greater force is applied to one side or the other the animal will turn in that direction. The automatic pilot has both a speed-up and a slow-down system which, when they work at equal strength, produce a level of alertness which matches the needs of normal, everyday, life.

When things slow down, as you sit in a comfortable chair beside a welcoming fire and watch television, for example, the *slow-down* branch takes over. Your blood pressure falls, heart rate is normal, you breathe slowly and easily, and your food is digested efficiently.

If life begins to get hectic, however, the *speed-up* branch assumes control. Heart rate and blood pressure increase, your digestion may be disturbed, and you could begin to perspire more freely. These changes are brought about by means of chemical messages acting under instructions from the ANS. The best known of these is the hormone adrenalin (in the United States it is known as epinephrine) sometimes termed 'jungle juice' because of its crucial role in the *fight or flight* response. That 'kick' in the pit of your stomach when you have been startled is due to extra adrenalin being released into the blood stream on the instructions of the 'speed-up' branch of the ANS.

'Fight or flight' in action

Imagine you are walking down a deserted street as night starts to fall. Suddenly a man emerges from a doorway a short distance ahead. He is carrying something in one hand and, in the failing light, it looks like a club.

While your 'thinking' mind is trying to decide exactly what the object is and how you ought to respond, the ANS has sounded the alarm signals and instantly sent your body into action stations. You experience instant alarm-startle followed by symptoms of anxiety.

Then the man passes under the light from a street lamp. You recognize him as your neighbour and see that he is holding nothing more menacing than a rolled-up copy of the evening paper! Orders from the ANS bring in the *slow-down* mechanism and, gradually, your heart stops racing, your breathing becomes regular and shallow again, you no longer sweat.

Alternatively, suppose the alert was not a false alarm. The man really is carrying a stick and he approaches menacingly. You decide to flee and run flat out into the busy shopping arcade and the safety of a crowd. Once again, with the moment of danger passed, the *slow-down* mechanism sets about the task of restoring things to normal and, although you may feel a bit shaky for some while after your escape, anxiety gradually declines.

The panic spiral

Many phobics report that their difficulties began with a panic attack. Some will explain that this attack came 'out of the blue' and was especially terrifying because they just could not think what was happening to them – or why.

I have already described some of the factors that make a person more vulnerable to this sort of attack. In a typical case the thoughts, the feelings, and the physical reactions will all occur within the space of just a second or so. But now we will slow down events to identify each stage of what has rightly been called the *panic spiral*.

In the last chapter we looked at the case of Susan who developed a phobia about railway platforms. Now let us see just what happened on that fateful evening as she stood by the platform's edge, reading her evening paper as she waited for the train that would take her home.

It was a routine activity she had carried out thousands of times before. But tonight would be different. As she turned a page, Susan happened to glance at the live rail. The sight triggered a memory. Perhaps she had recently seen an account of somebody falling to their death. She may have read the story without giving it more than a passing thought. But the item was stored away and now that glimpse of the live rail brings it into that part of her brain concerned with survival. The message was terse but urgent . . .

LIVE RAIL . . . DEATH . . . THREAT

. . . her automatic pilot reacted instantly. It was not concerned with where the supposed danger might be coming from nor with assessing whether or not the threat was a real one. Those tasks are performed by other areas of the brain, and these were still occupied with the newspaper story.

All Susan's ANS had to do was to alert her body for *fight or flight*. Adrenalin was released from glands located above her kidneys. In less than a second it was circulating in the blood, taking its message of alarm to every part of her body. Up to this point, Susan's attention had been focused on the paper. But the increase in adrenalin was immediately noted by her 'thinking' brain, which reacted accordingly. Why had the ANS ordered arousal? Where was the danger? What was about to happen?

The sudden concern was interpreted by the ANS as a need for still more arousal. Doubt and worry always strengthen the speed-up part of the system. Susan was aware of feeling suddenly, and inexplicably, afraid. The fact that she could not understand the reason for her fears only increased them.

Her heart began to thump wildly. Her mouth went dry. She felt sick and giddy. Fearful thoughts intensified the *fight or flight* response. The swiftly rising physical anxiety led to ever more panic-stricken notions. Forcing herself to move, Susan fled from the station.

From the first glimpse of that live rail to the moment when she ran off the platform, only a few seconds had passed. But in those moments of unreasoned and unreasonable terror, Susan's life had been drastically altered.

6
Before You Make a Start . . .

At this point in the book there may well be a number of important questions in your mind about this self-help training programme. So, before we move on to the course, I would like to devote a few pages to answering the queries most often raised by clients.

How long does the programme take?

There is no set time period for the training and you should proceed at a pace which suits your particular circumstances. Avoid the temptation of going too quickly in your eagerness to overcome the phobia. Never move on to a new stage in the programme until you have mastered the skills taught in the earlier ones.

For the first two or three weeks you should set aside about forty-five minutes per day, if possible doing some training *every* day. By the end of this period, basic skills should have been acquired and the programme will be less time-consuming.

Regular practice is very important. Shorter sessions carried out daily are far more effective than longer periods of training carried out irregularly.

Should I stop taking prescribed drugs?

If your doctor has prescribed tranquillizers or anti-depressants you should *continue to take them* while working on this programme. As you become less anxious and more confident your dependency on drugs for staying calm or warding off depression will begin to decline.

At this point you should consult your doctor, explain that you are following a behavioural programme which includes relaxation training, and ask for advice on how gradually to reduce your dosage. But you should not make any such changes except under the guidance of your GP or psychiatrist.

Are tranquillizers helpful to phobics?

In the short term, tranquillizers can be very useful when an anxiety problem first develops, as they make it easier for you to cope with life. But, after you have been taking them for a few weeks, the brain's chemistry readjusts to compensate for their 'damping down' effects.

This means that if you suddenly stop taking them, you are liable to suffer withdrawal symptoms and feel even more anxious than before. The withdrawal effects are minimized by gradually phasing out the drug under medical supervision.

Is special equipment needed for the programme?

Your body contains all the specialized equipment required for this training.

However, some people find it easier to learn how to relax if they can listen to the instructions on a cassette, rather than read them from a book. Details of my relaxation training tape can be found at the end of the book. In order to use this you will, of course, require a cassette recorder.

Will I find the programme upsetting?

Not in the slightest. There is absolutely nothing in this self-help course that is going to cause you any pain or distress.

Clients are sometimes fearful of embarking on a training programme because they imagine they might be forced to confront their worst fears right away. There is a procedure called *flooding*, or *implosion-therapy*, in which the sufferer is forced to confront the things they most fear, in a situation from which no escape is possible. As you can imagine, this leads to very intense anxiety. But the point is reached where the body is incapable of feeling any more afraid and so the fear begins to diminish. In this way the phobic comes to associate not feeling fearful with the previously feared stimulus.

Flooding can be helpful if you need to overcome your phobia very quickly. For example, a teacher who was a needle phobic wanted to work overseas and needed certain injections before she was able to travel. Time was short so her therapist suggested flooding. It was effective and enabled her to receive the necessary shots within a couple of hours of starting treatment. But this procedure is only suitable for certain types of phobia and should only be carried out under expert supervision.

In this programme you will never experience more than very slight, and perfectly manageable, anxiety.

Can even long-term phobias be helped?

This training programme should enable you to overcome even the most intense and deeply-entrenched phobias. However, you must realize that if you have been phobic for many years you will have become very practised at feeling and behaving in a particular way. Remember, a phobia is a *learned* response and, as with any learning, the more you practise the more skilled you become. Skills which have been perfected in this way are described by psychologists as 'internalized'. In such cases the reactions come automatically. There is no need to stop and think about what you are going to do next.

When you first learn to drive a car, each move has to be worked out in advance. Should I change gear now? How far should I depress the clutch? How fast should I take that corner? Once motoring skills have been internalized, however, all these activities become second nature. An experienced motorist can drive confidently and safely through rush-hour traffic while concentrating more on the problems of the day than on the road ahead.

It is the same with a phobia. If you have been practising your phobic response over a period of several years then it is likely that you will have got into the habit of feeling anxious and avoiding the fear stimulus. Even well-established habits can be changed, but it naturally takes time to learn new ways of reacting.

Your new skill – of being able to cope confidently and easily with the things which now make you feel so afraid – must be practised carefully and conscientiously if it is to replace your present behaviour.

Can my partner help?

If you are fortunate to have a partner or close friend, who is willing to help with this programme, then your training should prove easier and more enjoyable. I will be explaining exactly what other people can do to assist you at different stages in the programme itself.

The right kind of support is especially valuable if you are suffering from a very restricting difficulty, agoraphobia for example. Agoraphobics, in particular, often depend on other people to a very great extent. This dependency can quickly become a habit for both the phobic and her, or his, partner.

So, just as a phobic quickly gets into the habit of responding with fear and avoidance to certain situations, so can their partner, family, and often their friends as well, get used to responding to *them* in a particular way.

Ask your partner to read this book, and to pay special attention to those parts of the programme written especially for them. Discuss your programme with them and get help with planning and carrying through each stage.

If your partner is neither sympathetic nor prepared to be helpful, perhaps you have a relative or friend who can provide regular support. You will find it far easier to practise and perfect the skills taught in this book if there is somebody around who will take an interest and offer you encouragement.

Part Two

The Six-Step Training Programme

This part of the book should only be read after you have gone through Part One and understand how and why phobias develop. The purpose of this introduction is to describe the procedures taught in the six-step programme and to explain their significance.

Let's begin by going over the key points made in Part One:

1 You now know that a phobia is not an illness but a learned response.

2 You also know that the anxiety which is triggered in you by a fear stimulus is perfectly normal and natural. Under different conditions the arousal, or instant response which occurs as the speed-up branch of your autonomic nervous system takes control, could help save your life.

3 The reward provided by avoidance – and the resulting reduction in anxiety – has created the habit of avoidance.

4 The SAAR sequence establishes, and can spread, the effects of a phobic response.

5 Positive thinking which is unrealistic does not work. It only makes matters worse.

6 When forced to confront the cause of the phobia a 'panic spiral' can easily develop as negative thoughts increase physical symptoms. These distressing bodily changes lead to feelings of helplessness, confusion and fear.

With the problem so clearly stated the solution becomes equally clear. We must reverse the original learning process so that, instead of triggering fear, the same situations either arouse no needless anxiety at all, or else produce whatever positive feelings (pleasure, happiness, excitement) may be appropriate under those circumstances. For example a restaurant phobic or a social phobic should not simply be able to eat in public, or go to parties without fear. They should enjoy themselves!

Step One: Relaxation — the anxiety antidote

At the start of this book I explained that unrealistic positive thinking – where you tell yourself, very firmly, that you will *not* feel afraid – is worse than useless. When confronted by those things you have *learned* to fear you *do* become anxious, and because that reaction is directed by your automatic pilot, it is no use telling yourself to 'calm down' or to 'stop being so stupid'. Indeed, such thoughts often increase anxiety even more by emphasizing your inability to cope.

How then can control be exerted? Think back to my comparison between the two branches of the ANS and the use of the reins on a horse. Imagine that a clumsy rider has jerked on the left rein by mistake. His mount is now charging off in the wrong direction, but the error can easily be corrected by pressure on the right rein. When the speed-up system causes an unnecessary anxiety reaction it can therefore be brought back under control by strengthening the power of the slow-down mechanism.

There are two effective ways in which this can be done. The first is by eating. By encouraging digestion which, as we have seen, is controlled by the step-down portion of the ANS, the bodily reactions are reduced.

Thinking back to the comparison with a warship steaming into action, it is as if the Captain ordered his men to leave the guns and start cooking lunch, baking bread and laundering shirts. With nobody left to fire a shot no battle became possible! The trouble with eating your way out of anxiety is that you soon add extra inches to your waistline – which is one reason why over-anxious people are often rather overweight.

The second method is to learn relaxation. This is the body's natural antidote to anxiety since it is impossible to be both tense and relaxed at the same time.

In Step One of your training programme you will learn how to relax all the major muscle groups very deeply. I will then teach you to carry out quick relaxation, which achieves a good level of relaxation in a fraction of the time. You will also discover how to remain far more relaxed while going about your everyday activities.

Once these simple procedures have been mastered you have the ability to switch on the relaxation response anytime anxiety arises. By catching the panic spiral at a very early stage, controlling those sudden anxiety reactions becomes far quicker, easier and more certain.

Step Two: Creating your own programme

While relaxation is the key to successful anxiety control, it must be used correctly in order to prove effective. The procedures must be used correctly and in a structured way. If you simply learned how to relax, and then exposed yourself to those things which you fear most intensely, it is likely that you would still become very anxious. This is because too much anxiety is being generated for the relaxation response to deal with. The power of the body's *speed-up* commands is such that you cannot strengthen the *slow-down* system enough to overcome them.

You will be able to cope, easily and confidently, provided you raise the level of anxiety *gradually* while exercising careful control over your physical and mental responses. We can compare this to the approach that must be adopted when taking a hot bath. Step straight into the steaming tub, and you will recoil in discomfort from the heat. By first getting into water which is comfortably warm, and then, little by little, running in more hot water, you acclimatize your body to the heat.

The psychological equivalent of this gradual temperature increase is called *progressive desensitization*. By far the most effective proce- dure yet developed for the treatment of phobic anxiety, it involves overcoming your fears in gradual stages.

You begin with situations that can be dealt with reasonably easily, then slowly but surely progress to tasks which, at the start, seemed to be far more difficult. When you reach them, however, they appear no more difficult to cope with than those you confronted so effectively early on in your training.

In Step Two you will learn how to create a training programme exactly right for your particular phobic difficulty.

Step Three: Fantasy training

Before tackling the things you fear in real life, you will be taught how to confront them in your imagination. This fantasy training is helpful in two ways. First of all it allows you to reduce still further any anxiety which may arise when you start working through each activity in your programme. Secondly, it enables you to include situations which it might be very hard to practise in any other way.

Public-speaking phobics can imagine they are addressing large audiences, for example, and blood phobics can see themselves coping with physical injuries.

There are ways in which all these situations can, at least to some extent, be experienced in real life and you will be shown how this is done in Step Four. But fantasy training offers an easy and agreeable means for a very reliable method for defusing initial fears.

Step Four: Real life training

The only way to overcome a phobia is to confront things which you have previously avoided in real life.

By adopting a carefully controlled approach to these challenges, however, one can ensure that a small amount of anxiety is produced. By combining real life exposure with relaxation, and the confidence-building procedures taught in this part of the programme, you can train your body to associate once feared situations with self-assurance instead of fear.

Step Five: Coping with set-backs

Nobody ever learns any new skills without suffering at least some set-backs and disappointments.

If you have learned to drive a car, try to recall those early lessons. Almost certainly there will have been days when everything went perfectly and you were convinced you had finally grasped all the skills needed to pass the test with ease. But at the next lesson you ground the gears, jerked the clutch and stalled the engine. Embarrassing as they undoubtedly were, these mistakes did not mean you had mysteriously lost all the driving ability you showed a short time before. They simply indicated an 'off-day'. By not losing either your confidence or your nerve you were quickly able to regain that earlier level of excellence.

It is the same on this training programme. There will be days when everything seems easy and you are delighted by the progress being made. But inevitably there are also going to be occasions when you seem to be slipping back, occasions when what was tackled easily a few days before suddenly seems a lot harder to handle.

By preparing for such minor disappointment and frustrations you can come through them with your motivation and your self-confidence as strong as ever.

Step Six: Living without fear

With your phobia well on the way to being defeated, you can start looking forward to a life free from needless anxiety and unnecessary fears. Planning for this new life is important because how you face up to the future has an important influence on the chance of your remaining 100 per cent phobia free.

In the final part of the programme I will be giving advice on how to safeguard your physical health, combat depression and enjoy restful sleep.

This, then, is the shape of the training course you will be following over the next few weeks.

It is a self-help programme that has enabled thousands of phobia sufferers to overcome their fears. But, ultimately, *you* are the only person who can get rid of your phobia. Your doctor cannot do it for you, neither can a psychologist or a psychiatrist, the local hypnotherapist or the parish priest.

I cannot do it for you either. All I *can* do is to provide the knowledge you will need and the skills you must acquire. These are the basic raw materials from which a life without phobias can be created.

This book *cannot* help you if it is read but not acted upon, or if it is only acted on partially or in a half-hearted manner.

It *cannot* help if you go back to your old avoidance responses.

But . . . it certainly WILL help if you work at the procedures and start putting your new skills into practice.

And it *will* help if you are prepared to be patient, and work, *really* work, at the training programme.

Make a contract with yourself

The basis of any important commercial deal is of course, the legal contract, which states the contribution to be made by each party and what they can expect to get out of it. Contracts are often used in therapy too, not to bind the parties legally but to set down clearly and unambiguously what therapist and client intend to achieve during their time together, what each will contribute and what each can expect from the other.

Such contracts are useful because they focus attention on the agreed treatment goals. If, later on, there is any uncertainty about what the therapy aimed to achieve, those involved can settle the dispute by referring to the contract. You are going to be your own therapist because this is a self-help programme. Even so, you might find it very helpful to have a contract with yourself.

To state, at the outset, exactly what you hope to achieve and what you are prepared to do in order to attain those goals. From time to time, especially if your motivation seems to be flagging, refer back to this contract.

I have prepared a suitable therapy contract form for you. All that needs to be done is to copy it out (to avoid marking the book) and sign it.

Keep the contract where you can see it easily – perhaps you could pin it up on your bedroom wall – and glance at it every now and then. If your partner, or a friend, has agreed to help you, why not get him, or her, to sign the contract as well. That way both of you have a specific commitment to the process of change.

It will remind you of your feelings and intentions when the programme started and could provide that little bit of extra motivation which can sometimes mean the difference between going forward or giving up.

CONTRACT

I..................................sincerely wish to fight my phobia and win.

I will work through each step in this self-help training prog-ramme carefully and practise the skills I need to overcome my fears.

I will not be discouraged by occasional set-backs because I know these are likely to occur.

I will not seek excuses for putting off my training sessions.

I will make time – not just find time – to learn and use the procedures.

Date......................

I.....................am willing to help...............over-come..........phobia.

I will read the appropriate parts of the training programme and offer support and guidance as required.

Date......................

1

Relaxation – The Anxiety Antidote

When we were very young we were able to relax quickly and easily. You have only to watch a child asleep, or see the way an infant takes a minor tumble, to realize just how relaxed their bodies are. As we grow older, however, the stresses of life produce an increase in unnecessary muscle tension and – often without our even realizing the fact – our ability to remain relaxed slowly declines.

We can compare the results of such persistent stress to the effects of noise on people living close to an airport or a motorway. They soon grow so used to the deafening roar of jet engines or rush-hour traffic that the din is no longer even noticed.

We respond to bodily tensions in much the same way. After a while tension becomes so familiar we no longer notice it. We fail to realize that our 250 facial muscles are frequently set in a taut mask to help hide our feelings. We are unaware of the tense, awkward posture which places the muscles of neck, shoulder, and back under such a strain that they start to ache and throb. But there is another, equally important, consequence of this unnecessary tension. Within every single one of our muscles, from the largest and most powerful to the smallest and most delicate, is a complex arrangement of sensors whose task is to monitor their performance. These sensors respond to changes in tension and stretch, sending the brain information about the position of each part of the body in space. They also keep a check on the amount of effort being used to carry out everyday tasks.

If we attempt any task so far beyond our physical capabilities that the body might be damaged – lifting too heavy a weight for example – the sensors alert the brain that muscles are getting overstretched and we bring the activity to a halt.

Anxiety and the sixth sense

This little-known inner sixth sense – scientists call it the *kinesthetic system* – is the most vital of all the senses. Many people have triumphed over blindness or deafness, and even the loss of such sensations as taste, touch, or smell can be overcome. But if we were to lose our sixth sense, life itself would no longer be possible.

Where anxiety responses are concerned, feedback from this system plays an extremely important role. As the speed-up branch of our automatic pilot gains control, one of the effects is to tense key muscles in preparation for 'fight or flight'. This additional tension is immediately detected by the sensors and a warning is passed to our brain. Awareness of increased tension raises our level of alertness.

This greater arousal, feeding back into the muscles via the ANS, causes a further rise in bodily tension. And so the tension – arousal – tension sequence is repeated, again and again, forming an important component of the panic spiral. We run because we are afraid, but our fear increases because we run!

When the major muscle groups are already under needless tension your arousal threshold is automatically reduced. Picture two tumblers filled with water to different levels – one almost empty, the other almost full. Now imagine a small extra amount of liquid being poured into each. The almost empty tumbler takes up the extra liquid easily. The nearly filled glass overflows.

It is the same with bodily tension. If you are already highly stressed it requires only a small amount of additional tension to trigger an anxiety attack. If you have ample reserves, because those muscles which do not need to be under tension are relaxed, then extra stress can be absorbed without difficulty.

The first skill you will have to master, therefore, is that of relaxation. This involves not so much learning as *relearning* since you will be rediscovering an ability possessed in full measure during childhood, but mislaid in the process of growing-up. Over the next few weeks you will acquire *three* different forms of relaxation.

DEEP RELAXATION is designed to banish tensions entrenched in your muscle groups. By reducing the amount of unnecessary anxiety arousal, Deep Relaxation will ease away the stress which creates pain, improve your sleep and – perhaps most important of all – lower your overall level of anxiety.

RAPID RELAXATION Once you have learned how to relax deeply, mastering this second skill is fast and simple. Rapid Relaxation enables you to banish unnecessary tension in less than a minute. You will find this skill especially helpful on any occasions when anxiety levels start to rise.

ACTIVE RELAXATION Finally you will learn a third skill, the ability to keep non-essential muscles completely relaxed while performing everyday activities, even when these are especially strenuous such as jogging or playing tennis.

Deep Relaxation

Time required

To master Deep Relaxation set aside two twenty-minute periods a day for 7–14 days. After that time you can reduce the sessions to one twenty-minute period a day for the next 7–14 days.

Exactly how long it will take to acquire this skill varies from person to person. You should not start to learn Rapid and Active procedures until you have been practising Deep Relaxation for at least ten days.

Best time

By carrying out your relaxation training first thing in the morning and last thing at night you enjoy the added benefits of preparing yourself for the day ahead and winding down just before you go to sleep. This should ensure a more confident and less tense approach to life and improve your night's rest.

Where to relax

You will need a quiet room which has a bed, couch, or comfortable armchair. Some people prefer to darken the room slightly by drawing the curtains.

Using the instructions

Before your first session read the instructions below several times. When you feel you have remembered most of the major muscle groups, and how to relax them, have a short practice session during which you work briefly through each group in turn.

Do not worry if, at first, you find it hard to recall all the actions required. This will come after just a few sessions. Alternatively you may find it easier to tape record the instructions. If you decide to do this be sure to speak quietly and clearly. Make the recording in a quiet place so that the tape does not contain any crashes or bangs which might startle you. Talk slowly, allowing plenty of time to carry out each set of movements before describing the next stage. As already mentioned earlier I have made such a recording as part of a cassette course on agoraphobia. You can obtain free details by writing to the address at the end of this book.

How to begin

Before embarking on your first session of relaxation training make sure you can enjoy an entirely uninterrupted twenty minutes. Take your phone off the hook. Make sure your children realize you must not be disturbed.

If your partner is agreeable, and you feel that company would help you relax more easily, then why not carry out these sessions together. You do not need to suffer from a phobia to experience great benefit from the mastery of these skills. Almost everybody in today's pressured society is suffering from needless bodily tension, as figures for deaths from coronary heart disease show only too clearly. Relaxation helps reduce the everyday stresses of home, family and workplace. It combats 'free-floating' anxiety (that is anxiety not triggered by anything in particular), improves one's sleep, and enhances physical health.

Before you start, remove or loosen tight clothing, and take off your shoes. Begin your relaxation training as follows . . .

1 Lie back on the bed, couch or chair. Place your arms by your sides, legs uncrossed and stretched out in front of you.

2 Keep your lips lightly together, jaws loose and tongue resting at the bottom of your mouth. Smooth out your brow and let your eyelids gently close.

3 For a few moments simply lie still and feel yourself sinking deeper and deeper into the chair or on to the bed.

4 Now take a long breath. Try to breathe in for a *slow* count to 8. Breathe out again, just as slowly, while counting backwards from 8 to 1. Repeat this *four* times.

Each time you breathe out I want you silently to repeat the word – *relax*. Every time you tell yourself to 'relax' focus on the feelings of letting go and unwinding. As you say the word to yourself, picture worries and problems, your fears and physical tensions being expelled from the mind and body on each breath of exhaled air.

After lying quietly and comfortably for about one minute you can start on the first in a series of exercises designed to train your body to notice the difference between tension and relaxation.

To do this, each muscle group is first deliberately tensed before being allowed to unwind as completely as possible. Each step of this exercise can easily be recalled by means of this simple phrase . . .

A Soothing Feeling – My Body Has Peace.

The first letter of each word stands for one of the six major muscle groups you will be working on in turn.
These are:

A – arms and hands
S – shoulders and neck
F – face (forehead, eyebrows, muscles around the eyes)

M – mouth (jaw, lips, tongue, and throat)
B – body (chest, stomach and buttocks)
H – hips (thighs, calves and ankles)

Finally we have:

P – pictures in the mind which soothe away mental stress.

We start, then, with muscles in the arms and hands.

A group – fingers, wrists, forearms
You tense these muscles by clenching your fists as tightly as you can. Squeeze the fingers tight . . . tighter . . . tighter still. Press them into your palms. Now hold that for a slow count to 5.
  Feel the tension . . . feel the tension. Now relax. Open your fists. Stretch out your fingers and let your hands flop back against the bed or chair. Notice the difference between tension and relaxation in the muscles. Now move to . . .

A group – upper arms front
You tense these muscles by bending your arms at the elbow and attempting to touch your shoulders with the back of your wrists. This tenses the biceps, the muscles at the front of the upper arm.
  Hold and feel that tension during the same, slow, count to 5. Let go. Drop your arms and let them rest lightly against the bed or chair. Notice, as before, the difference between tension and relaxation. Now move to . . .

A group – upper arms back
You tense these muscles by straightening them as hard as you can to tense the tricep muscles, the large muscles at the back of the arm. Hold for the same slow count to 5 and then let your arms flop down. As the tension flows out of them notice what it feels like to allow these hard-working muscles to unwind more and more deeply.

You have now relaxed the first major muscle group and should take a few moments to rest quietly and to focus on your hands, wrists, and arms. Your breathing should be quiet and regular. Each time you breathe out, imagine any tensions still remaining in the arms flowing out of those muscles, emptying them entirely of stress.
  Next turn your attention to those parts of the body so often affected by needless muscle tensions resulting in aches and pains – your shoulders and neck.

S group – shoulders

You tense these muscles by shrugging your shoulders. Draw them up as high as you possibly can so that tension builds and builds. Hold and feel that tension for a slow count to 5. Drop your shoulders. Allow them to flop down and unwind.

Notice, as before, the difference between tension and relaxation in these muscles. Now move to . . .

S group – the neck

You tense these muscles by pushing your head back firmly against the bed or chair. Hold the position for a slow count to 5 while feeling the build-up of tension. Let go . . . flop out the muscles. Allow your head to rest gently against the support.

With the second major muscle group unwound, take a few moments to focus on this part of the body while you lie still and quiet, breathing in a rhythmic and shallow way. Each time you breathe out repeat the word 'relax' and, as you do so, feel any remaining tension being eased gently away from your neck and shoulders. Now move to the muscles of . . .

F group – the face

You tense these muscles by frowning as hard as you can and squeezing your eyes tightly shut. Hold for a slow count to 5. Feel the tension building up. Now let it all go. Relax the muscles around your eyes. Allow the lids to rest lightly together. Notice the difference between tension and relaxation in your eyebrows and in the muscles around the eyes.

Next, tense the muscles in your forehead and scalp by raising your eyebrows as if in surprise. Notice the build-up of tension for the slow count to 5. Relax. Smooth out your brow. Keep your eyes looking straight ahead. Feel the tension flowing away from your face.

M group – mouth (jaw, lips, tongue and throat)

You tense these muscles by pressing your lips tightly together, clenching your teeth, pushing the tip of your tongue against the roof of the mouth. Hold for the slow count to 5. Relax. Let the tension flow away from these muscles and notice the difference as they unwind and relax.

Once again take a few moments for general relaxation. Make sure your breathing is slow and regular. Each time you breathe out say the word 'relax' to yourself. Focus on the muscles of the face and mouth. Feel any remaining tension slipping away.

B group – body (chest, stomach and buttocks)

You can tense all these at once by doing the following. Take a very deep breath. Really fill your chest with air until the tension in the muscles around the ribs and in the diaphragm is considerable. At the same time flatten your stomach as much as you can. Draw in the muscles and pull towards your spine. While doing these two actions squeeze your buttocks tightly together. Hold for the usual slow count to five.

Now expel the air from your lungs. Release the tension in the stomach muscles. Let your buttocks relax. Allow the muscles to flop out so that needless tensions simply melt away.

The final muscle groups to work on are those of the hips and legs.

H group – hips (thighs, calves and ankles)

You tense these muscles by straightening your legs as much as you can, pointing your toes downward. Hold for a slow count to 5. Relax . . . allow the muscles to unwind as completely as possible as you rest your legs against the bed or chair.

Complete the physical relaxation part of your session by spending a full minute focusing first on the muscles of the body and legs, then on *all* the muscles which you have been relaxing.

Notice any remaining tension and imagine it flowing easily from your muscles. Keep your breathing shallow and regular, silently repeating the word 'relax' each time you breathe out, and imagining all the tension flowing from your body as you do so.

Before we go on to look at ways of relaxing the mind as well as the body, it will be helpful to summarize the sequence of exercises in this training session.

1 Work through the major muscles in turn. The memory jogger – **A** Soothing Feeling – **M**y **B**ody **H**as **P**eace – will help you remember the sequence to follow.

2 Tense those muscles in the way described.

3 Hold for a slow count to 5.

4 Release the tension rapidly and allow the muscles to unwind. Notice the difference between tension and relaxation.

5 After each set of muscles has been tensed and relaxed spend a few moments focusing your mind on that part of the body. Keep your breathing slow and shallow, repeating the word 'relax' each time you breathe out.

6 Move to the next set of muscles and repeat the procedure.

Now relax your mind

'P', the final letter in our memory jogger, reminds you to ease mental as well as physical tensions. After working through all the muscle groups you should lie still and quiet, breathing in a slow, rhythmic manner and focusing your attention on the key word 'relax' each time you breathe out.

Now start to develop a mental picture of any image which helps you feel at peace. Some people like to imagine a colour, perhaps a rich purple or a warm yellow, which makes them feel at ease and content. Others prefer to picture a place they know well. Somewhere, perhaps, where they spent an especially happy period of their lives.

But your scene does not have to feature somewhere which really exists. The joy of working with mental images is that you can create a world known only to you where there is no pain or danger, no sadness or suffering, in which you can feel only pleasure, security and a deep tranquillity. At the end of each relaxation session you can then travel to this secret place and refresh mind and body in its soothing surroundings.

You may wish to escape into a countryside setting, or perhaps you prefer a warm beach by a clear, green-blue sea under a cloudless sky. Whatever image you select build up the scene as vividly as you possibly can.

Suppose your choice is for sun, sand and sea. You might picture yourself stretched out on the soft, golden beach of some tropical island. The air is filled with the scent of wild flowers. Close by, the palm fronds stir gently in the breeze. A calm, clear ocean laps the bay gently beneath an azure blue sky.

See these images in your mind's eye. Feel the warmth of the sun on your body and the soft firmness of the beach beneath your back and legs. Stretch out one hand and let the warm grains of sand trickle through your open fingers. Listen to the sounds of the sea, the muted cry of birds, and the soft rustle of the trees. Smell the clean, fresh air, the saltiness of the sea air and the perfume of brilliant wild flowers which fringe the peaceful bay. This is your personal, private, unspoiled paradise. A unique kingdom of tranquillity which only you can ever enter and enjoy. There you feel completely safe, happy and content.

At first these images may not be very complete and you might find it hard to hold them for more than a few moments. But if you persevere it will become easier and easier to build and sustain a mental scene so powerful that it embraces and enchants all the five senses. Hold this image for five minutes or so (longer if you wish) at the end of each session. Then open your eyes and stand up *slowly*. Try to carry feelings of mental and physical relaxation into your everyday life.

Six tips for successful relaxation

1 Keeping your eyes lightly closed throughout the session will help shut out distractions.

2 Focus all your attention on the muscle group being relaxed. At first there may be a tendency for your thoughts to wander, but if you gently but firmly return your mind to the task at hand such lapses in concentration will grow less frequent.

3 Never try to force yourself to relax since this will simply make you more tense. Allow feelings of relaxation to develop naturally. Once this has happened take a few moments, between working on each group of muscles, to relax more and more deeply. Silently repeating 'relax' to yourself serves the same purpose as a *mantra* in transcendental meditation. It trains your mind to associate a particular feeling – relaxation – with a key word.

4 Always try and hold your training sessions in the same room, and if possible at the same time each day. By doing so you will get into the habit of feeling more relaxed whenever you enter those surroundings. In this way it becomes easier and quicker to master the skill. When you are practised you can, of course, relax with equal ease in almost any surroundings.

5 As you start to relax you may feel a slight chill. This is perfectly normal and shows that the slow-down branch of your ANS is starting to take control.

6 Never get up with a rush or move away in a hurry after relaxation. Not only will this make the session less beneficial but you could also feel slightly giddy. If you do, there is no cause for alarm. Merely sit still and the dizziness will quickly pass.

Using a timetable

As some people find it easier to follow a written training schedule I have included a timetable in Part Three. This indicates which stage of the programme you might have reached by a certain time and provides space on which to keep notes. You should copy the outline on to a separate sheet of paper and keep this somewhere convenient for easy reference. If you find yourself working slightly more slowly – or more rapidly – than this timetable suggests, do not feel concerned. Everybody learns these procedures at a different pace. The important thing is never to move to a new skill until you have gained some experience of those that precede it.

After carrying out two twenty-minute sessions of deep relaxation for 7–10 days you may well be ready to master the new skill of Rapid Relaxation.

RAPID RELAXATION This should be carried out five or six times each day, but you can – if you like – replace *one* of your deep relaxation sessions with this new procedure. It only takes about thirty seconds to complete. But, with only a little training, you will find it possible to use this method to relax quickly and easily under almost any circumstances.

Begin as follows... Sitting in a comfortable chair you should tense *all* the muscle groups at the same moment.
Do this by:

1 Clenching your fists hard and bending your arms at the elbows, trying to touch wrists to shoulders.

2 Pressing your head against the chair.

3 Squeezing the eyes tightly, clenching the teeth and pressing your lips together firmly.

4 Pushing your tongue against the roof of the mouth and frowning hard.

5 Hunching your shoulders, taking and holding a deep breath.

6 Flattening your stomach as though anticipating a blow.

7 Straightening your legs and raising your ankles from the floor.

8 Hold the tension in all these muscles for a slow count to 5.

9 Now flop out completely. Try to imagine your body as a length of elastic which has been stretched as taut as possible and then allowed to snap back.

10 Collapse into the seat like a puppet whose strings have suddenly been cut through.

11 Feel the tension flowing from those muscles like water pouring through a swiftly opened sluice gate.

12 Take slow, shallow breaths and, as you breathe out, silently repeat the word 'relax'.

Carry out four or five sessions of Rapid Relaxation at other times of the day as well. Use the procedure whenever you start feeling slightly anxious, before tackling anything which presents a special challenge and following stressful encounters.

After a while – exactly how long will vary from person to person – it will be possible to relax rapidly but deeply *without* actually having to tense and release the muscles. Your mind and body will be trained to respond to the word 'relax' by letting go of needless tensions.

When this point is reached all you need do is sit or lie comfortably, arms by your side and legs uncrossed, and repeat the key word 'Relax' a few times. Almost immediately you will start feeling less mentally and physically tense. Taut muscles will unwind and anxious thoughts disappear, to be replaced by a sensation of calm confidence.

After practising both Deep and Rapid Relaxation for 7 – 10 days you can begin to acquire the final skill – Active Relaxation.

ACTIVE RELAXATION You can use this in any situations in which you need to remain calm while performing some physical activity. After one of the Deep Relaxation sessions remain sitting or lying still. Open your eyes and look around the room while keeping the rest of your body motionless. Feel what it is like to be observing your surroundings while everything except your eyes remains motionless.

Next, keeping the rest of your body still, slowly turn your head to study every detail in the room. Notice the furnishings and the decor, the ornaments and the pictures. You may turn your head as much as you like provided your body, arms and legs stay still.

Now stop moving your head and start talking to yourself. What you actually say is unimportant. Recite a poem, read out an imaginary shopping list, tell yourself a funny story. The purpose of this exercise is simply to practise using the muscles required for holding a conversation while the rest of your body remains deeply relaxed. As you talk, try to notice the difference between those muscles controlling the jaw, tongue and neck which are now under tension, and the remainder which should feel entirely free from unnecessary stress. After a few moments stop talking, close your eyes, and relax totally for a while.

When you are ready to proceed, open your eyes once more and start moving your arms around while ensuring that the rest of your body stays quiet and relaxed. Bend your elbows, twist your wrists, waggle your fingers, swing your arms from the shoulders. As you make these movements, notice the difference between the tension in muscles being made to work and those allowed to remain relaxed.

After a while let your arms drop back to your sides and relax for a few moments. Now, slowly stand up and start walking around the room. Do not hurry or move jerkily. As you walk notice the tension in your legs and compare it with the feelings of relaxation which should still be present in your torso, shoulders, neck, face, arms and hands.

After walking around for a minute or so return to your bed or chair and relax again for a couple of minutes. Complete the exercise by spending a few minutes enjoying the feeling of deep mental and physical relaxation.

When you have become more confident of your ability to keep one part of the body relaxed while another is hard at work, increase the range of activities performed. Introduce Active Relaxation into your everyday life.

You can start using this form of relaxation while doing physically demanding work, when walking, jogging or taking part in a sport, or when gardening or driving your car. You will find that all types of activity can be carried out more easily, more enjoyably, and with greater success if *only those muscles directly involved* are kept under tension. Active Relaxation also helps to *lower* your anxiety threshold because needless tension has been eliminated.

Making relaxation part of your life

At first you will have to tell yourself to relax whenever anxiety or tension seem to be building up. Only when the skill has been well mastered will relaxation become an automatic response to stress. But this is true of *any* new skill. Think back to learning to drive a car, to take part in a sport, or to cook a meal. When you began it was essential to pay close attention to the task in hand. Only after the skill had been *internalized* could you use it effortlessly and to maximum effect.

The more you practise relaxation the faster this skill will be perfected. The more *regularly* you practise the easier it will be to achieve complete relaxation. The better your relaxation skills, the easier it will be to reduce anxiety at source, to prevent the panic spiral from developing and to deal quickly and effectively with situations which give rise to fear.

Summary

Procedure	*Time required*
Deep Relaxation	Two twenty-minute sessions per day for between 14 – 21 days.
Rapid Relaxation	Carry out 5 – 6 sessions, each lasting approximately 30 seconds. Start after you have been working with Deep Relaxation for 7 – 10 days.
Active Relaxation	One session per day for 7 – 10 days.

Only start working with a new relaxation procedure when you feel confident of having mastered the one before. In the meanwhile, however, you should read the next chapter (Step Two) in which I explain how to create your personal self-help training programme.

2

Creating Your Own Programme

Although a great many people will be experiencing the same sort of phobic difficulties as yourself, each person's phobia is still – in a very real sense – unique. Unlike a physical disease, such as measles or mumps, where the causes and consequences are universal, the phobic experience must, inevitably, differ in some important ways from one person to the next.

The manner in which your fears first developed, the extent of the restrictions they now impose, the intensity of response to feared situations, and the ways you have found for coping with this disability, remain highly personal. They arise from the whole of your life's experiences and, for this reason, will never be exactly duplicated by anybody else.

This means that, although every self-help programme based on the procedures in this book will follow the same general pattern, the precise content of each will vary according to an individual's particular needs and special circumstances. Your programme will, therefore, be created by you for your own personal use.

Understanding your fears

In order to design and monitor such a programme it is necessary to understand, as clearly as possible, the physical and mental responses your phobia produces and the conditions under which anxiety arises.

You may believe, especially if you have lived with your fears for many years, that you already have this knowledge. It is more likely, however, that your insight is actually rather limited and perhaps not especially accurate. This is hardly surprising since everybody, phobic or non-phobic, experiences their strongest emotions in a highly subjective manner.

As a result, people with phobias are often only able to describe their feelings in a fairly vague and rather general way. For example:

'I stepped out of the house and was overcome with fear. I wasn't able to move at all for a few minutes. I was sure I would faint if I did.'
Agoraphobic, aged 26.

57

'Going to work on the train I suddenly became panic stricken. I had to get out at the next station. I felt sick and was trembling.' *Travel phobic, aged 19.*

'I heard on the weather forecast that we would have thunder storms in our area and felt terrible. I didn't know what to do I was so afraid.' *Thunder phobic, aged 57.*

'I have been terrified of vomiting all my life. I have not been sick for twenty years but this is no comfort. I only think: "It's got to be me next." I am so afraid that if my children are ill I shall catch it.' *Vomit phobic, aged 39.*

Such comments are typical of the way in which most phobic anxiety is described. While this may be sufficient to provide a general understanding of the problem, more comprehensive information is necessary in order to create a satisfactory training programme.

The Record Diary

The starting point for constructing your programme is to obtain detailed and comprehensive information about the way you behave when confronting situations that cause anxiety. This is the only way to achieve an accurate understanding of exactly what makes you afraid and how your fear is expressed. To do this you will have to observe your own behaviour in a detached and objective manner.

In Part Three you will find the format for a Record Diary in which these notes can be kept. I suggest you copy the headings into a pocket-sized notebook that can be conveniently carried around. This will enable you to write down the information required as soon as possible after each event.

Record Diary information forms an important part of your training programme because it provides great insight into the precise nature of your fears. The notes also allow you to monitor your progressive improvement as the phobia starts to disappear.

Information in the Record Diary should be collected under the following *seven* headings:

1 *Before I start*
Under this heading write down all the thoughts which come into your mind before you tackle anything that arouses anxiety. Note what you say to yourself, the way you feel and how you assess the likely outcome.

Typically such comments tend to be fairly negative:

'I shan't be able to cope . . .'
'I shall feel faint . . .'
'I will probably have a panic attack . . .'
'Everybody will be staring at me . . .'
'I'm no good in these situations . . .'

Do not worry if your remarks are, like those quoted above, generally unhelpful and liable to undermine rather than enhance self-confidence. As you work through the programme it will be possible to change these so that you take an optimistic, yet at the same time entirely realistic, view of what will be happening.

2 *What . . . when . . . where . . .*
In the second column you record *what* you were doing, or attempting to do, *when* you were doing it and *where* it was being done.
To make sure that these notes are as complete as possible, be certain to include details of:

(i) Time and place.

(ii) People present. Who they were (friends, strangers, colleagues, employees, superiors, etc.), how many there were, their attitude (friendly or distant, kind or critical, helpful or hostile), and what they were saying or doing.

(iii) What you were doing, or attempting to do.

(iv) The physical conditions – was the place hot or cold, dusty or damp, humid or windy? Were there any objects or animals present that had some relevance to the way you felt? Do not be concerned if your entries under this heading are rather sparse at first. It may be hard for you to remain in the situation long enough to take in many details, and anxiety adds to the difficulties of making clear observations. With a little practice, however, this task becomes fairly straightforward.

For example, an early entry in the notes of a bus phobic read:

'8.35am. Monday. Got into bus. Doors shut . . .'

At this point he became so frightened it was impossible for him to pay attention to anything more until the next stop where he hastily left the bus. Ten days later, however, he was able to record:

'8.35. Wednesday. Sat on nearest seat to self-closing doors. Bus crowded. Pushed against window by large person on seat next to

59

me. Roads wet and slippery. Rather misty. Hot and muggy inside bus. Bus seemed to go very fast, lurched on the bends . . .'

Although he felt just as anxious and only made two stops of the journey it was possible for him to become sufficiently detached to notice and recall what was going on around him.

3 Physical feelings
Under this heading you will note how your body responded to the challenges. Did your heart rate increase? Was your mouth dry? Did you feel sick or giddy, trembling or faint and so on?

4 Mental feelings
Under this heading note the thoughts in your mind during the activity. Were you able to think clearly or did you become confused? Were you telling yourself how 'dreadful' the situation was and how you could not possibly cope any longer?

Record all that you can remember of these thoughts, and do so as soon after the event as possible.

5 What was good about the situation?
So far you will probably have been noting mostly negative feelings. But the situation may actually have had a few positive aspects to it, even if you could not fully appreciate them at the time.

For example, a travel phobic noted:
   'Pleasant breeze blowing through partly-opened window . . .'
   'Feeling of relief at sitting down after standing at bus-stop.'

A woman with agoraphobia commented . . .
   'Sun warm on face . . .'
   'Spring flowers in the park very beautiful . . .'
   'Displays in store windows interesting . . .'

Initially, you may find it impossible to see anything good in your situation. But do not give up. After a while you will almost certainly be able to find a few positive features to note down.

6 Afterwards
Note down how you felt immediately after the event. What thoughts are uppermost in your mind? Are you angry with yourself at not having remained calmer? Are you depressed because, yet again, you were forced to abandon an activity? Are you thinking miserably that your worst fears were fully realized?

7 *Anxiety rating*

In the final column rate your anxiety, using a number from 1 to 6, according to the amount of anxiety aroused.

If you felt calm, confident and happy when carrying out the activity, rate it – 1

If you felt slightly apprehensive but generally coped in a calm, confident way, and mostly enjoyed the experience, then you should rate it – 2

If you coped well, but experienced neither anxiety nor pleasure when carrying out the activity, rate it – 3

If you felt some anxiety but managed to continue with only a slight loss of confidence or ability, rate it – 4

If you felt very anxious and found it almost impossible to remain in the situation, although you somehow managed, then rate it – 5

If you were so frightened that you had to abandon the attempt entirely, then rate it – 6

Recording intense or occasional phobias

It may be that your phobia is very intense and restricting or is caused by something which occurs only occasionally in your life. For example, somebody severely disabled by agoraphobia may never venture out of doors at all. A vomit phobic might go out of his (or her) way to avoid having to deal with sickness. An air phobic could become afraid no more than once or twice each year when flying abroad on holiday with the family. Under these circumstances records should be kept as follows:

1 While working through feared situations – both in your imagination and in real life – later on in this programme.

2 On any occasion when you are obliged to confront the things which make you afraid.

For example, an air phobic should be sure to write up the Record Diary as soon as holiday plans start being discussed. Entries could include – looking at holiday brochures, going down to the travel agents to book the tickets, driving to the airport, waiting in the departure lounge and so on.

Start keeping your Record Diary from today onwards and continue making careful and thorough notes throughout the training programme.

Now set a goal

The next stage in creating your programme is to establish some clear goal. This must be an activity you would like to be able to carry out entirely on your own. That is, without a partner standing close at hand, or hovering in the background.

It is important to define this goal clearly and precisely. Saying that you want to 'get out more'; 'not feel afraid of dogs'; 'eat in public'; or 'make a speech' leave too many questions unanswered.

Where do you want to go when you 'get out more'? How large a dog would you like to approach without fear? Do you want to eat with friends or with strangers, in the company canteen or a cosy restaurant? Is your speech to be made to a small group of colleagues or a large audience of strangers?

For a person with agoraphobia, specific goals might be: 'Walking to the school to meet my children;' or 'shopping in the local supermarket.'

For a dog phobic: 'Stroking a medium-sized, friendly dog'; or 'Being able to enter a room in which there is a large dog.'

For a restaurant phobic: 'Eating with friends in a crowded restaurant'; or 'Having a meal with one other person in a quiet restaurant.'

For a public speaking phobic: 'Giving a short talk to a group of colleagues in a small conference hall' or 'addressing an audience in a large hall.'

The precise nature of your initial goal will, of course, depend entirely on the nature of your phobia and the kind of restrictions it imposes on your life. Someone suffering from agoraphobia might consider it far more important and rewarding to meet her children from school than to go shopping in town. So she would start by working towards this goal. Once it had been achieved she could then work towards achieving the second goal, then a third, and so on.

Similarly, a restaurant phobic could be more attracted by the idea of being able to enjoy a quiet meal with an intimate companion than dining with friends in a crowded room. The public speaking phobic might have a more urgent need to address a group of colleagues than to talk to a large group of people.

So establish an overall goal which has relevance to your current life. Choose something you would really like to be able to do, that you would enjoy, and that would produce some positive rewards by its attainment.

Now turn to Part Three. Copy the Progress Chart on to a sheet of paper, following the design shown, and write your overall goal in the top left-hand space. You may feel able to do this right away. Alternatively, you might wish to keep the Diary for a week or ten days, in order to arrive at a suitable goal.

The next stage is to work out a number of sub-goals that will enable you to progress, slowly but surely, towards that major accomplishment. Start by thinking of something you are confident of being able to carry out, with only a small and quite acceptable level of anxiety. As a guide this would be something that rated around 4 on the Diary's anxiety scale.

Write this in the bottom space of your Progress Chart. Now think of an activity that might cause you slightly more anxiety (5 on the scale) and write this in the next space up. Continue in this way until you have eight or ten sub-goals between your present position and the activity you wish to carry out.

These tasks can be compared with stepping stones across a wide river. The skill is to place them at just the right distance apart to allow you to cross as fast and as safely as possible. If they are too close together progress will prove needlessly slow.

This first list should only be regarded as provisional, since you may well find it necessary to change some of the sub-goals in the light of experience. If progress seems too slow you will want to develop a slightly more ambitious list. If you are experiencing too much anxiety then you should consider introducing additional sub-goals. But remember, it is very important to experience some anxiety in each situation. Only by doing so can you learn to cope with these feelings.

As illustrations of completed Progress Charts, here are two created by Mary, who was suffering from agoraphobia, and Caroline, who was a dog phobic.

Mary's Progress Chart

When working out her training programme, Mary selected as her overall goal – 'shopping at the local supermarket, buying goods from counters a long way from the exits, and waiting in a queue to pay at the check-out.'

Her list of activities read as follows:

1 Walk to corner of street, wait and return home.

2 Walk to bus stop and wait for five minutes.

3 Catch bus, travel one stop, and walk home.

4 Travel two stops by bus and walk home.

5 Travel to town centre and catch bus home.

6 Go into town, enter supermarket and look around without buying anything.

7 Go to supermarket on quiet day and make purchases from counters near entrance.

8 Make purchases from counters further from entrance.

9 Make purchases from counters close to entrance when shop is busy.

10 Make purchases in all parts of store on Saturday afternoon when it is busy and probably necessary to queue at the check-out.

In practice, Mary found it too difficult to progress from 5 to 6 on her list. So she introduced an extra activity into her programme:

5a: Stand outside supermarket looking in through windows.

But she also discovered that, having gone inside the supermarket she felt sufficiently confident to make purchases from counters quite some way from the exits. This meant that she was able to move straight from 6 to 8.

Caroline's Progress Chart

When collecting information about her phobia, Caroline carried out various experiments to see how much anxiety was aroused by different types of encounter with dogs. She found that small, leashed, dogs seen in the open air aroused the least fear. Large, unrestrained dogs in confined spaces were – she knew – the most fearsome.

Her overall goal was to be able to stroke a medium-sized, familiar, and friendly dog in a medium-sized room. With the co-operation of a dog-owning friend she created, and then carried out, the following list of activities:

1 Looking at small, leashed dog at a distance and in the open.

2 Approaching the same dog more closely.

3 Coming within touching distance of the dog.

4 Touching the dog on the back quarters while animal is held by owner.

5 Stroking the dog on the head.

6 Approaching same dog when unleashed.

7 Stroking unleashed dog.

8 Being in large room with leashed dog.

9 Being in medium-sized room with leashed dog.

10 Touching leashed dog in medium-sized room.

11 Stroking dog, unleashed but held by owner in room.

12 Stroking unleashed and unrestrained dog in room.

Notice how Caroline gradually progresses from just looking at a dog under the conditions she knew would produce only a small amount of anxiety (small, leashed, in the open air) to being indoors with the same dog.

By working towards her overall goal in this way, and using the relaxation and other procedures which will be described later in the programme, she had no difficulty in entirely overcoming her phobia. The list of goals was, in fact, reduced in practice as she found that she could move without difficulty from 4 to 7 and then from 7 directly to 10.

Phobias — simple and complex

Where there is a single fear stimulus (e.g. spider, dog, cat, bird, bridge, hair, thunder, insects) – these are sometimes described as *monophobias* – there may only be one overall goal. That is, to pick up a spider, pat a dog, stroke a cat, watch birds, cross bridges and so on. Once that target activity can be accomplished without undue anxiety, the phobia no longer presents any problems.

More complex, multiple, phobias usually have more than one overall goal that needs to be achieved before life returns to normal. Along the target activities of a person suffering from agoraphobia, for example, one might find:

1 Meeting my children from school.

2 Visiting the dentist.

3 Going to church, the theatre or cinema.

4 Shopping in a supermarket.

5 Travelling on holiday unaccompanied.

6 Riding on a bus or train.

Each represents a different target which must be worked towards, independently of the others. You should find, however, that when one or two of these goals have been attained, the others can be accomplished far more quickly and easily. This is partly because you now have greater experience in using the procedures involved in a self-help programme. But an equally important factor is a general reduction in anxiety levels which comes about when one major source of stress has been overcome.

Start by selecting the most meaningful goal, perhaps in consultation with your partner, and then work towards that. Only when you are well on the road to success here should you embark on a different training schedule intended to attain a second goal. Proceed in this methodical way until all your goals have been attained.

Summary

1 Start collecting information about your phobia using the type of Record Diary illustrated in Part Three.

2 Keep notes under the 7 headings listed and try to write them up just before and immediately after any activity which arouses anxiety.

3 Be sure to note down any positive features in the activity, in addition to all your more negative thoughts and feelings.

4 Identify some activity which you would very much like to accomplish calmly and confidently. Choose something which is truly relevant in your life as this will increase motivation.

5 Write this overall goal at the top of the chart.

6 Devise a list of activities (sub-goals) which lead you, slowly but surely, towards accomplishing that goal.

7 Start with some activity which arouses an anxiety rating no greater than 4 on the Diary scale.

8 No activity should make you more fearful than this when the time comes to tackle it.

If you do start feeling more anxiety than is comfortable, revise your Progress Chart to include further intermediate activities. Equally, you can drop some of the sub-goals, if you are making better progress than anticipated.

Multiple or complex phobias usually involve a number of different overall goals each of which must be achieved before anxiety difficulties are completely resolved.

When you have been practising Deep Relaxation for 10 – 14 days and can create a good visual image at the end of each session you will be ready to move to Step Three (Fantasy Training) of the programme. Meanwhile remember to write up your Record Diary and to work out the programme's overall and sub-goals. These should be entered on the Progress Chart.

3

Fantasy Training

Because avoidance has helped create your phobia, the only way to eliminate these difficulties is by learning to confront and cope with situations which make you anxious. Experience has shown that it is far easier to do this in real life – Step Five of the programme – if you first work through each activity in fantasy.

By imagining yourself coping calmly and successfully with things that currently arouse anxiety, you both build your confidence and develop the habit of remaining relaxed, rather than fearful.

Fantasy training also has the advantage of allowing you to work through activities that would prove complicated or costly to arrange in reality. An air phobic, for example, might go through an entire flight, in his mind's eye, without having to wait for an opportunity to practise in real life.

It must be understood, however, that Fantasy Training is not an alternative to going through a particular activity in reality, but is a preliminary step along the way.

Time required

Set aside fifteen minutes per day for your fantasy sessions, which are best held immediately following Deep Relaxation.

Fantasy training in action

Start with the first activity on your Progress Chart, that is the one which can be carried out with only a slight amount of anxiety.

After relaxing physically, spend a few minutes unwinding mentally by picturing that quiet and peaceful scene.

Now switch from those soothing images to the first situation on your Progress Chart. Keeping your eyes lightly closed and your breathing shallow, imagine yourself, as vividly as you possibly can, carrying out that activity in real life.

Take your time – each session should last no less than fifteen minutes – so that you are able to develop the images slowly, carefully and with as much attention to detail as possible. Try to see yourself performing the task confidently and without apprehension. When unwanted thoughts and ideas start distracting you, simply notice that your mind has wandered from the task at hand, and gently return your attention to the activity being practised.

Creating vivid mental images and holding them in the mind's eye is a skill which takes some while to master. You will find it easier to sustain a lengthy and detailed scene as you go along. But, again, do not become worried when distracting ideas intrude. Do not dwell on these intruding thoughts, just observe they have arisen before directing your mind back, calmly but firmly, to the training task.

Some people, while finding it difficult to create clear and detailed visual images are still able to imagine themselves performing the activity very clearly. Do not feel concerned, therefore, if this is the way your own imagination prefers to work.

Should you find yourself becoming too anxious, switch off the scene and return to the pleasant, relaxing, images which you use at the end of each relaxation session. Use the muscle exercises to banish physical tension and the pleasant scene to eliminate unhelpful thoughts. When the anxiety has subsided return to the task.

Even when thinking about a particular task in a very detailed manner, it is still likely you will complete it faster in the imagination than would be possible in real life. If this happens you should simply go over the scene again and again until the full training session has been completed.

When the time is up, relax for a few moments by returning to your peaceful images, before getting up slowly and returning to your everyday activities.

Creating detailed images

The more realistic your fantasy scenes, the more effective this part of the programme will prove when it comes to reducing anxiety in real life. Information from your Record Diary should be used to add realistic details to the scenes you create in your mind's eye.

Try to involve all five senses in your creations so that, as described above, you not only see and hear what you imagine to be happening but also experience the sensations of touch, taste and smell.

If the scene involves leaving home, for example, you might start by picturing yourself putting on your shoes and coat. While doing so, you would try to 'feel' your shoes as you put them on. You would also 'notice' the texture of the cloth and the weight of the material as you push your arms into the sleeves of the coat. You would then picture yourself walking to the front door and opening it wide, feel the doorknob under your fingers, hear the sound as the handle turns and the door opens, and sense the breeze on your face as you step outside.

Do not worry if your early images are brief and lacking in details. This is perfectly normal since most people find fantasy training a skill that takes time to perfect. Each situation must be imagined three times on separate days before you attempt it in real life.

Key points to remember

* You must imagine yourself carrying out each activity *alone*.

* You must repeat each task in your imagination during one daily session on each of *three* successive days.

* Each fantasy session must last at least fifteen minutes. The longer you spend imagining yourself carrying out each activity, the more rapidly you will learn to cope with anxieties in real life.

* After each training session make a tick on your Progress Chart. Notice that, if the programme is followed correctly, these ticks will form a diagonal line across the chart.

* Create images which are as vividly realistic as possible and involve all five senses.

* If you feel anxiety rising too sharply, switch off that scene and return to the pleasant mind relaxer. When you feel calm again return to those images and try again. Should anxiety persist after a number of attempts it means that the Progress Chart must be modified. The sub-goals are too far apart and you must introduce some intermediate stages between the last activity you tackled and the one you are now attempting to cope with.

* Keep notes on these sessions in your Record Diary, filling in details under each of the 7 headings.

Summary

Procedure   *Time required*

Fantasy Training   One fifteen-minute session per day following
                     Deep Relaxation. Start with first activity on
                     your Progress Chart and work gradually up the
                     list. Repeat each *three* times before going on to
                     the next.

At this point you should read Step Four and make any plans necessary for working through the first item on your Progress Chart in real life. But remember that you should only do so after first going through that situation *three* times in your imagination. Once the programme is fully under way, you can be rehearsing one task in your imagination while carrying out the earlier activity in real life.

Remember to note both fantasy sessions and real life training on your Progress Chart.

4

Real Life Training

Before moving to this Step in the programme, make certain you have completed the following earlier stages:

1 *Deep Relaxation*: This should have been carried out for at least ten days. You will now be able to relax deeply without too much difficulty and to create a peaceful and soothing mental image at the end of each session.

2 *Rapid Relaxation*: You should be able to use this procedure to relax quickly and easily.

3 *Active Relaxation*: Should have been practised on a number of occasions so that you are able to detect unnecessary tensions in muscles not being used directly for a particular activity.

4 *Record keeping*: You will have been keeping detailed notes about your phobic responses in the Diary.

5 *Goal setting*: You will have identified an overall goal and worked out a series of sub-goals by which this can be achieved. Both the target goal and the activities leading up to it will have been written on to the Progress Chart.

6 *Fantasy training*: You must work through each situation in your imagination, during a fifteen-minute fantasy session, on three separate days, before attempting them in real life.

The sequence of training sessions on a typical programme might, therefore, look like this:

DAY ONE
First *fantasy* training session with item *one* on the Progress Chart.

DAY TWO
Second *fantasy* training session with item *one* on the Progress Chart.

DAY THREE
Third *fantasy* training session with item *one* on the Progress Chart.

DAY FOUR
First *real life* training session with item *one*.
First *fantasy* training session with item *two*.

DAY FIVE
Second *real life* training session with item *one*.

Second *fantasy* training session with item *two*.

DAY SIX
Third *real life* training session with item *one*.
Third *fantasy* training session with item *two*.
DAY SEVEN
First *real life* training session with item *two*.
First *fantasy* training session with item *three*.

And so on . . .

Remember
* Never attempt an activity in real life until you have worked through it in your imagination.

* Complete each activity *three* times. First in fantasy and then in reality.

If you find it possible to cope with a certain activity in fantasy but still feel unacceptably anxious during the real life practice, then be prepared to revise your sub-goals. Anxiety greater than 4 on the Rating Scale suggests that you are attempting something too ambitious. Go back and look at the list again to see how you might introduce an intermediate activity.

For example, a travel phobic who found it too difficult to progress from travelling one stop by bus to travelling three stops, could simply get off at the second stop. Equally, a spider phobic who became over-anxious when trying to progress from approaching a small spider to a larger one should use a spider of intermediate size. I will be explaining later how such real life situations can be organized.

It is important to appreciate that levels of anxiety are also influenced by your overall emotional and physical condition. Most people experience mood swings from one day to the next and, for the phobia sufferer these emotional changes often produce feelings of confidence on some days and greater apprehension on others.

There will be occasions, therefore, when you feel capable of moving more quickly up the Progress Chart and of coping successfully with activities much further up the list. At other times, you could find that an activity which caused only very little anxiety the previous day, now makes you feel unexpectedly afraid. To safeguard yourself against these influences, work through the programme methodically. Do not be tempted to proceed too quickly on 'good' days or assume that you are falling behind and failing if you suffer an increase in overall anxiety on 'bad' days.

In Step Five I will be giving you advice on how to combat such ups and downs in order to ease your way through the programme. For the moment, however, bear in mind that you should only make changes in your list, either increasing or reducing the number of activities leading up to the overall goal, if you have found the task either far easier or far harder than anticipated during two of the three training sessions.

* Remember that it is essential to feel some *slight* anxiety in each of the situations being practised. Only in this way can you train your body to cope with that activity in a calm and controlled manner, as your automatic pilot gets into the habit of responding with slow-down instead of speed-up commands.

Real life training in action

Keep these six points in mind when starting to work through your activities list in real life.

1 Before each session, use Rapid Relaxation to eliminate unhelpful mental and physical tensions. While carrying out the task use Active Relaxation to strengthen the power of the slow-down system.

2 Note your thoughts and feelings in the Record Diary immediately before the session. On your return, fill in details under the remaining headings.

3 Identify training sessions with the letter 'T'. This enables you to monitor your progress both on the programme and in other areas of your life.

4 As in fantasy sessions, each activity should be carried out *three* times in real life before you move to the next on your list.

5 Tick the appropriate column on the Progress Chart when you complete the session.

6 Each session should last *at least* fifteen minutes.

Organizing special training sessions

With some types of phobia it is relatively simple to carry out a series of graded activities leading towards the overall goal. In agoraphobia, for example, progressive exposure usually means travelling further and further from home. Other phobias may require you to use your imagination and make preparations beforehand in order to complete some of the activities listed.

Caroline, the dog phobic, for instance, asked an animal-owning friend to co-operate in order to create specific situations for her real life training sessions.

Phillipa, a spider phobic, developed her training programme in collaboration with her husband and teenage son. Her overall goal was to be able to pick up a large spider in a tumbler and carry it out into the garden. As they lived in the country it was not difficult for her family to catch a variety of spiders. Her son also searched local toy shops for 'joke' spiders made of rubber and plastic.

The first item on Phillipa's training schedule was to remain in the dining room for fifteen minutes (remember this is the *minimum* period for each session) while a *small* toy spider was placed on the table some ten feet from where she sat. Over the next twelve days, Phillipa gradually came closer to the table by moving her chair nearer, a foot at a time. She practised at each new distance on *three* separate occasions before decreasing the distances between her and the spider.

The next stage was for Phillipa to touch the toy spider. She did this, over a period of nine days, by gradually placing her hand closer and closer to the toy. The small spider was then replaced by a larger, toy one. Phillipa found she could cope with only a slight amount of anxiety when standing six feet away. Once again she came closer and closer until she was able to touch the large toy.

The process was then repeated using a small, living spider in a jam-jar. After further training she was able to touch the jar containing this animal and, later on, found herself able to pick up the jar without distress. A slightly larger spider was then introduced. Finally, Phillipa progressively approached the bath in which a large, garden spider had been placed, and was able to remove it in a glass.

Her training schedule had a total of thirty sub-goals which she worked through over a three-month period. At no time did she feel more than slightly apprehensive and, by the end of the programme, her fear of spiders had disappeared.

'I can't say I actually like them', she admits, 'but if I find one trapped in the bath I have no hesitation in catching it in a glass and liberating it unharmed in the garden. Before, I would simply have screamed and fled, no matter how tiny and insignificant the spider was.'

Now let's look at another phobia, a fear of flying, which also required prior arrangement. For years, Alan and his family had been unable to take their holidays very far from home due to Alan's intense fear of travelling by air. His phobia had also delayed promotion in his company since senior managers were expected to fly on several business trips a year.

The early items on Alan's training schedule presented few difficulties since they only involved visits to travel agents, studying brochures on air holidays and organizing tickets. Nor were later stages of his programme hard to arrange. He took two weeks holiday and spent half-an-hour each day at his local airport. He watched aircraft take off and land, listened to announcements of departures and arrivals, and generally became used to the atmosphere of the small, but busy, airport. He also tape-recorded announcements and used these to add realism to his fantasy training sessions. While at the airport Alan practised Active Relaxation.

The next step was slightly – but only slightly – harder to organize. He wanted to practise sitting relaxed and at ease in an actual aircraft. A letter to the airport manager and the public relations department of the main carrier produced immediate results. He was given permission to spend time inside a fuselage mock-up used for training air stewardesses. Later he went inside stationary jets on the tarmac.

Alan was able to practise relaxing in the actual seats. He also carried out some fantasy training while inside the plane, imagining himself flying off on holiday with his wife and children. He had tape-recorded the sounds of aircraft taking off and played these, through phones, as he sat in the stationary aircraft. Finally, he reached a point where it was possible for him to take a short, domestic flight.

'I still am no great fan of flying,' he acknowledges, 'but at least now I can travel on holiday and take business trips for the firm without any real apprehension. The phobia, which had been with me for at least twenty years, was completely overcome during the four-month period.'

If your training programme requires special facilities, never be afraid – or ashamed – of writing to people who can help you to make the necessary arrangements. You will find most of them sympathetic and prepared to help with the facilities needed.

Restaurants are usually prepared to let public-eating phobics practise sitting at a table in a relaxed and confident manner during periods when they are normally closed to customers. Theatres and cinemas will usually lay on similar facilities for agoraphobics. Bus companies, the railways, and airlines can also be persuaded to help with your programme.

So do not restrict your training activities because you think that something will be impossible to organize. Seek the help you need and only revise your schedule after exploring all possible avenues. Here are some more suggestions for ways of developing training tasks:

Blood phobics can use stage blood (available from fancy-dress suppliers and joke shops) to have different kinds of 'wounds' created on volunteers.

Public speaking phobics can practise delivering short talks to groups of relatives or friends. This can be done at home to start with. As the training proceeds try to address audiences in larger halls. Ask your local school or college for permission to practise on their premises at times when their class or lecture rooms are not in use.

Aggression phobics can ask friends and relatives to 'role play' different characters in dramas where gradually-increasing amounts of assertion are required.

Interview phobics can rehearse different strategies, again with relatives or friends playing the part of the interviewer.

Thunder phobics can tape radio weather forecasts of storms (perhaps with help from a partner or friend) and create their own training cassettes using sound effects records, which can be obtained from most large record shops.

Bird or insect phobics can use a variety of stuffed animals or realistic toys.

Be creative when developing your real life training sessions and do not be afraid to involve others in your programme. Many individuals and organizations are prepared to assist, once they understand your requirements.

How WASP helps

Whenever you are carrying out an activity in real life, keep the word WASP in mind. It will help you remember to stay calm and relaxed.

WASP stands for WAIT – ABSORB – SLOWLY PROCEED.

WAIT! Avoid hurrying. The faster you go the more likely it is anxiety will arise.

ABSORB! Take in your surroundings. Pause and look around you. You may be surprised at how interesting even familiar surroundings can become.

SLOWLY PROCEED! Carry out the task slowly. Never rush.

This is the opposite to the way most phobics cope with the things they fear. The main idea racing frantically through their minds is: 'I must get this over with . . . I must get away . . .'

As I explained in Part One, such thoughts serve to increase confusion and raise levels of arousal, so fuelling the anxiety and making a panic attack more likely. WASP will help you stop running, mentally or physically, through the encounter.

So, if anxiety starts increasing, try to stay where you are. Use Rapid Relaxation to bring your speed-up system under control. And WAIT!

You feel anxious when you step on to a bus, train, or plane. You feel anxious as you rise to speak to a group. You feel anxious as you walk down the street. You feel anxious as you see a spider, or a dog, or a bird.

Your first impulse is to escape and avoid as quickly as possible. Do not do so . . . WAIT!

Use Active Relaxation as you sit down, as you stand before the audience, as you walk towards your destination, as you watch the animal you fear. Give your slow-down system time to regain control.

As you WAIT, take in details of your surroundings. Make mental notes for later use in your Record Diary. Do not simply stand or sit motionless with your eyes blinded and your ears deafened by anxiety. Absorb the sights and sounds around you. Notice details large and small. Observe what is happening, what the weather is like, what sort of window displays there are in shop windows, whether the trees are in leaf, what other people look like. ABSORB everything.

SLOWLY PROCEED. Move in a relaxed and controlled manner. After a while pause again, not because you have felt a spurt of anxiety this time, but simply to 'stand and stare'. Allow your body to experience feeling in control of the situation instead of out of control.

You may experience some little difficulty in doing this at first, but this is perfectly usual. When one has got into the anxiety habit it takes time and practice to learn new ways of responding. But such changes will come about as you work through the training programme.

How other people can help

If you are the partner, relative or close friend of somebody suffering from a phobia, there is a great deal you can do to help.

Start by reading this book so that you understand how these anxiety problems arise and what can be done to overcome them. You might also take up my earlier suggestion of going through relaxation training with your partner (from now on I shall refer to all those closely associated with a phobic as their 'partners') as this can help to sustain motivation. The skills you master will, of course, help you to get rid of needless tension and so combat stresses more effectively.

Phobias, especially ones which greatly restrict the sufferer, are often sustained by the things which others do, usually with the best and kindest of intentions. The problem is that depending on others can quickly become a habit.

Discouraging this dependency may be difficult. The partners of people with a severe phobia often regard them as invalids who need 'looking after'. If the partner has treated the phobic in this way over a long period, then the phobia sufferer's habit of depending on them will be matched by the habit of being depended upon. It must also be recognized that such dependency can provide certain rewards for the partner.

The more any activity is avoided the stronger the fear which surrounds any attempt to confront that task. As the partner of a phobic, here's how you can help most effectively.

Six ways to enhance the programme

1 Do not *immediately* withdraw your assistance and insist that the person 'face up' to his, or her, fears. This would be both cruel and counter-productive. Instead, as new activities are tackled successfully, you can simply stop performing that particular task.

For instance the partner of someone with agoraphobia may have got into the habit of going down to the local shops when household supplies run low. Once the point in the programme has been reached where it is possible to call at those shops, the partner should stop shouldering this particular responsibility. But he, or she, should continue their usual assistance in situations not yet dealt with during training. This might mean, for instance, going on doing the weekly shopping at the supermarket – or continuing to accompany your partner during such trips.

2 Involve yourself in the programme right from the start. Work with your partner to decide on overall goals which you both agree would be useful. But remember that he or she must have the final say in what targets are to be set. Discuss the sub-goals and help your partner to decide where the programme should start.

3 Continue to encourage and support your partner during the training. Make a point of asking what has been accomplished each day and show your pleasure at progress made. Look at the Progress Chart and Record Diary, perhaps offering *constructive* comments about some of the entries. Give a small gift (it does not have to be costly) whenever a key target is achieved.

4 If set-backs occur, and they are almost inevitable during the course of a programme, try not to become impatient or irritated. Instead, work with your partner to see how the activities list might be modified to overcome the obstacle. Do not complain when progress seems slow or patchy as such swings in mood are perfectly normal.

Be on the lookout for 'excuses' not to practise an activity. Wet weather, a headache, being 'too busy', not feeling 'in the mood' are just a few of the 'good reasons' why training should be put off until tomorrow. There may well be some truth in these statements but you should be firm and suggest that your partner tries anyhow. You should not, however, make a major issue out of it if they remain unwilling.

Instead work through the activities list together to see if some revision is needed. Read my comments on overcoming set-backs (Step Five) and see if any of those suggestions would be helpful. Always let the sufferer take the final decision however, since you should never pressure a person into doing something he, or she, really does not want to do.

5 If you are accompanying your partner when a panic attack occurs do not immediately return home.

Find somewhere to sit and rest, walk back a short distance, but try to remain close to the place where the anxiety arose. Avoid the temptation of constantly asking how your partner is feeling. Lengthy discussions about anxiety tend to make matters worse.

Talk about something else until your partner starts getting over the attack. No matter how intense it may be, the panic will subside in a relatively short while and, once gone, is unlikely to return for a considerable time. The crucial point is never to leave the situation until the anxiety has started to decline.

6 Fears which we cannot share, and do not really understand, can all too easily be dismissed as trivial or 'silly'. These views usually lead to a sense of irritation and the belief that the phobic could overcome his, or her, difficulties if only he, or she, would *try* a little harder. The reasons why such an attitude is both mistaken and unhelpful should by now be clear. The progress made in overcoming the phobia will depend, to a signficant extent, on your encouragement, and understanding.

Summary

Procedure	*Time required*
Real Life Training	However long it takes to complete the desired activity. This should not normally take less than 15 minutes. The longer you spend on the session (within reason) the more rapidly anxiety will decline. Start the first Real Life session after going through the first item on your list *three* times in the imagination.

Remember to write brief details in your Record Diary and to tick the Progress Chart. You should now read Step Five of the programme and use the procedures described if any set-backs or difficulties are encountered. •

5

Coping with Set-backs

As you work through the programme it is quite possible, although by no means certain, that you will experience a few set-backs and delays. There may be times when your progress seems to have come to a complete halt, or is far slower than you had hoped for. There may also be occasions when, after a period of great success, you suddenly get bogged down. At times like this it is only natural to feel a bit depressed and disheartened.

Maybe you will start to believe that you have failed, or assume that the programme is not working. Perhaps you will conclude that your phobia cannot be defeated. While understandable, such a response is not, of course, at all helpful, since it undermines self-confidence, reduces motivation and increases anxiety.

There are a number of reasons why such difficulties arise and in this Step of the programme I want to describe the three most commonly encountered problems, explain why they occur and tell you what can be done to resolve them.

Difficulty One – the sudden stop

The 'sudden stop' is well illustrated by what happened recently to one of my clients.

Having suffered from agoraphobia for many years Alice was making excellent progress and had, for the first time in a decade, travelled two stops by bus on her own. The next day, as she was about to set out for her second practice session, Alice suddenly became so anxious she found herself unable even to leave home. The following day she felt just as afraid. Far from continuing with her previously excellent progress she seemed to have come to an abrupt halt.

This block was all the more puzzling and disappointing because nothing had gone wrong during the bus journey. Indeed Alice had found it a surprisingly pleasant and interesting experience. She felt happy to travel so far from home, and returned delighted with herself. Why then should she have felt so fearful of repeating the enjoyable experience that she resorted to avoidance again?

There are two main reasons for such 'sudden stops'. The first is that an activity may have been too mentally and/or physically demanding. In Alice's case, she moved straight from: 'Standing at the bus stop and watching buses go past without trying to board one' to 'Boarding the bus, travelling two stops and walking home.'

This had involved a total of ten minutes on the bus and a journey home on foot of more than a mile. The task drained her both physically – she was not used to taking much exercise – and emotionally. Her condition the next day was rather similar to a person who, not having taken any strenuous exercise for ten years, decides to start jogging.

Instead of building up stamina slowly but surely, through gradually increasing the distance covered, while reducing the time taken, our keep-fit enthusiast decides to cover six miles in thirty minutes. At the time his body copes reasonably well but, next morning, every muscle is stiff and aching as a result of such unreasonable treatment.

Alice's body was protesting in much the same way and for the same reasons. Because she was more tired than usual, her mind was also more vulnerable to anxiety and depression. These feelings combined to lower her threshold to the speed-up response so that, when she became slightly anxious prior to setting off, the slow-down mechanism lost control.

To appreciate why Alice, and many other phobics, quite often become anxious, and experience a set-back, just as their programme seems to be having a good effect, we need to consider the second factor involved in the 'sudden stop'. This arises, paradoxically, not because the training procedures are proving ineffective, but because they are starting to work rather well.

In Alice's case, having triumphantly accomplished something she had believed was quite beyond her capabilities, a whole new world of freedom suddenly opened up before her. She now realized that it really might be possible to get rid of the agoraphobia which had restricted her life so severely for more than ten years. It was an exciting and stimulating prospect, but also a slightly frightening one.

We can best understand some of the conflict she experienced by thinking about the feelings of a person employed, for many years, in a tedious, routine, and dead-end office job. One morning, the manager brings some surprising news. As a reward for loyalty and hard work he is being offered promotion to area supervisor.

Now, in place of the familiar office routine he will enjoy a very varied and stimulating lifestyle. Instead of having to clock on at nine and off at five he can set his own hours. The promotion means he must travel widely and meet many new people. Each day will be slightly different from the last. Gone is that hated rut. Gone the office treadmill.

Opportunity beckons. To transform his life all he need do is accept the chance being offered. Does he take the promotion without hesitation? Perhaps – but not necessarily.

Maybe he reflects that dull routine is not really so bad after all. In a nine to five job at least he knows exactly what is expected of him, where he must be at a certain time and which tasks have to be completed within the working day.

This new job seems to have no such reassuring structure. It certainly offers fresh opportunities and the chance to expand his horizons, but it also threatens him with the possibility of unfamiliar difficulties and problems for which he may not have any answers. In mounting panic he thinks . . . How will I be able to cope? Will I be capable of meeting those new challenges? Will excessive demands be made on me? Should I take a chance, or stay with what I know?

It is the same when somebody suffering from a severely restricting anxiety condition sees the gates of their prison start to swing open. All of a sudden it becomes clear that, when the phobia disappears, so too will a way of life which – despite its pain and tedium – at least has the merit of being familiar and reassuring.

But – the sufferer asks – suppose the programme does work, as it seems to be doing, and the phobia is no longer a problem? What demands will be made on me by partner, family and friends? How well can I cope with these new challenges?

In Step Six I will be looking at ways in which you can plan your life ahead and putting forward ideas that will help the phobia remain defeated for ever. But how, in the short-term, can the 'sudden stop' be dealt with most effectively?

1 – Check the sub-goals
On the basis of prevention being better than cure, the best way is, of course, to prevent 'sudden stops' from occurring in the first place.

You can do this by making certain your list of sub-goals is not over-ambitious, and that the 'stepping stones' across the 'river', represented by each new activity on the Progress Chart, are not so far apart that you run the risk of falling into the water and being swept away.

2 – *Change the sub-goals*

If you do come to a sudden stop then examine the sub-goals and introduce one, or more, additional activities. In Alice's case this simply meant travelling one stop by bus on three separate occasions) before attempting two stops. This simple manoeuvre was sufficient to overcome the block entirely.

3 – *Think about your feelings*

It is only natural to feel afraid of the unknown. And by bringing about the changes involved when you rid yourself of an intense and restricting phobia you will be venturing into unfamiliar territory. Anticipate such fears, but do not let them get out of proportion.

You can and will be able to cope when the time comes. Never see your phobia as a refuge against the real world. It is not. It is an unnecessary and unhelpful response without which you will be much better off.

Difficulty Two – feeling anxious about not feeling anxious

There is an old story about a lodger who wore very heavy hobnailed boots. Every night, returning home late from the pub, he would sit on the edge of his bed, remove each boot in turn and let it fall with a crash to the floor. His landlady, who slept in the room underneath, was rudely awoken by the noise and complained bitterly to him the next day. Finally, she could stand it no longer and threatened to throw him out if her sleep was disturbed again.

That night he came back even later than usual, removed his right boot and dropped it with the usual deafening thump. Then, suddenly remembering her warning, he carefully took off the left one, placed it quietly on the carpet and fell asleep. Several hours later he was woken up by an anguished cry from the landlady. 'For heaven's sake,' she cried, 'drop the other boot!'

I am reminded of that story when clients describe this second difficulty to me, because they are in much the same position as that unfortunate landlady. They too are waiting for the 'other boot' – in the form of an anxiety attack – to drop. They are made anxious by the knowledge that they are no longer anxious, and this anxiety often triggers the very panic attack they feared.

As the training procedures take effect, it becomes relatively easy to do many things that were previously avoided. Instead of experiencing a high level of anxiety they find it possible to cope, even to enjoy, a widening range of activities. At this point some phobics begin to wonder, 'Can it last?' and to ask fearfully, 'How long before the next panic?' They tend to see themselves as the man who, having fallen from the fortieth floor of a skyscraper was heard to murmur 'so far, so good' as he hurtled passed a third floor window.

Negative thoughts arise such as: 'This can't last . . .' 'I am going to feel anxious soon . . .' 'It's too good to be true . . .' 'Tomorrow isn't going to be as easy as today . . .'

These undermine motivation and set up a self-fulfilling prophecy of failure. The most effective way of preventing such anxiety generating anxiety is through the use of 'Positive Self-Talk Statements' and 'Cue Cards'.

Learning Positive Self-Talk

I would like you to look at the entries made in your Record Diary under the headings – *Before I start* and *What was good about the situation*. Comments in the first category might include . . .

'I feel sure I cannot cope with the demands that will be made on me.'
'I will panic.'
'I am hopeless in this kind of situation.'

Remarks in the second category might mention such factors as . . .

Anything attractive or beautiful.
Anything stimulating or amusing.
Anything enjoyable or rewarding.

To create Positive Self-Talk Statements you combine items of information from these two headings. In order to be of value each has to possess three specific qualities:

1 It must relate directly to any difficulties you anticipate.

2 It must be realistic about the likely outcome.

3 It must contain practical advice about how each situation can be tackled successfully.

The best way of illustrating how such statements are constructed is to look at extracts from the Record Diaries kept by my clients.

Notes from the 'Before I Start' section in the Diary of a thunder phobic:

'I know there is thunder in the air. I can't stand the thought of a storm. I shall go mad if there is a storm close by.'
'I cannot cope with hearing thunder warnings on the radio.'
'The sky is leaden, terrifying. I feel sick with dread. I cannot work.'

What was good about the situation?
'Sound of rain on the windows and roof was soothing.'
'Awe-inspiring cloud formations.'
'Smell of the earth after a storm.'
'The dramatic way lightning dissolves the darkness.'

From these lists this lady was able to create the following Positive Self-Talk Statements. Notice how each satisfies the three conditions listed above.

Positive Self-Talk Statements:
'When a thunder storm breaks it is going to be hard for me to control my anxiety. It will help if, instead of listening out for claps of thunder I concentrate on the sound of the rain splashing against the window. This is soothing and agreeable.'

'The sky is very dark and menacing, there is going to be a storm which will make me distressed. But right now I shall concentrate on studying the sky. It really is very powerful and dramatic. The texture and colours are magnificent. I will focus all my attention on that feature.'

'The lightning flashes will be easier to watch if I notice the way the darkness is suddenly dissolved by the brilliant and beautiful blue light.'

Notes from the 'Before I Start' section in the diary of a travel phobic:

'The swaying of the bus, and the lurching as it stops, make me feel faint.'
'I cannot bear the idea of being pressed inside a crowd of people. I shall not be able to cope. I shall make a fool of myself.'
'There is no way I am going to be able to cope with a fifty-minute train journey. I shall be ill in the compartment.'

What was good about the situation?
  'Nice being able to close my eyes and relax in the bus after a hard day.'
  'Interesting to watch some of the other travellers on the Underground.'
  'Countryside looks very beautiful at this time of year.'
  'The breeze through the open window is pleasantly refreshing.'

Positive Self-Talk Statements:
  'I know that the journey by train will be difficult but I shall be able to deal with it by concentrating on the changing landscape.'

  'The movement of the bus is quite unpleasant but I shall be able to cope if I sit near the window, feel the breeze on my face and look at the passing scenery.'

You will notice that none of these examples include such blanket assurances as: 'I am going to cope . . .' 'I will not panic . . .' or 'I am not going to feel afraid.'

Although these comments may seem comforting when you start out they end up by being very false friends, for the reasons I explained in Part One. If you grow anxious they are immediately disproved, so your feeling of losing control increases.

  'I am not going to feel afraid . . .' is replaced by the thought
  'I *am* going to feel afraid.'
  'I am going to cope' can easily change into 'I am *not* going to cope.'

Avoid these dangers by anticipating that *some* anxiety will arise – indeed if you do not feel a small and controllable amount of anxiety then you must revise the training programme to make the situations slightly tougher. You can only get into the habit of coping with mild anxiety by experiencing it. Your Positive Self-Talk Statements should, therefore, begin with something along these lines:

  'I may find this rather difficult but I shall cope more easily if I remember . . .'
  'The situation may be tricky to handle at times, but it will prove less difficult if I . . .'
  And so on.

To summarize this procedure, let's look at a set of Positive Self-Talk Statements prepared by an agoraphobic to see how they satisfy the three conditions outlined above:

1 They must relate to specific difficulties.

Correct: 'I may find it slightly hard to cope at the start of a storm but I will keep anxiety under control if I study the texture and colours of the clouds.'

Incorrect: 'It may be hard but I shall cope somehow.' (Notice that this does not relate to any specific feature of the difficulty, nor does it offer any practical advice about what to do if anxiety levels start rising.)

2 They must be realistic about your chances of success.

Correct: 'Walking down to the shops will make me slightly anxious but . . .'

Incorrect: 'Walking down to the shops is going to be very easy for me.'

3 They must offer practical advice about how the problem may be tackled successfully.

Correct: 'Riding on the bus will be easier if I sit close to the window.'

Incorrect: 'If I sit near the door I can get out quickly should I panic.' (This is wrong because it incorporates a way of avoiding the situation.)

Continue to construct Positive Self-Talk Statements as you work through the programme. To remind yourself of them write the most appropriate ones out on small cards and carry these with you. These prompts are called *Cue Cards* and serve the same kind of function as the autocue device used by TV speakers to remind themselves of their lines. They help you remember important ideas for controlling anxiety even when you are under extra stress.

Cue Cards in action

In addition to writing down Positive Self-Talk Statements, your Cue Cards should also be used to remind you of any other hints and tips which will help make life easier. If you look at your Record Diary entries under the headings 'Physical and Mental Feelings', you will get a clear idea of whether a particular situation produces mainly bodily or emotional anxiety symptoms or both. Your Cue Card should then include comments under these headings, designed to help you remember what procedures to follow in order to bring these under control.

A public speaking phobic, for instance, noted that his worst anxiety occurred while waiting to speak. Physical symptoms included trembling hands, rapidly beating heart and a dry mouth. The mental symptoms were confusion, a tendency to forget the starting point for his talk and a sensation of unreality.

A restaurant phobic's diary produced the following information:

Situation: Lunchtime. Walking into busy restaurant with friends.

Physical feelings: Throat muscles so taut it is hard to speak or to swallow. Feel myself getting excessively hot. Mouth very dry. Feel sick.

Mental feelings: Cannot concentrate. Difficult to talk. Memory poor and forget what I wanted to say.

One of the Cue Cards prepared by each of these individuals is shown below as an illustration of the sort of advice that can prove helpful.

Cue Card prepared by a public speaking phobic:

Situation: Waiting for the moment to speak while being introduced.

Physical Feelings: 1 Use Active Relaxation when standing and talking. 2 Take a sip of water to moisten mouth before standing up. 3 Place hands on table or behind back to steady them. 4 Steady legs by resting lightly against the table. 5 Pause for a few seconds before starting to speak. 6 Do not rush.

Mental feelings: 1 Start by thanking chairman for introduction. 2 Introduce topic with reference to previous speaker. 3 Quote facts and figures from page 3 of notes. 4 Use visual aids. 5 Ask for questions.

Positive Self-Talk: 'This may be slightly tricky at first, but when I get warmed up my anxiety will decline.'

'I shall be able to control anxiety when starting more easily provided I do not rush.'

Cue Card prepared by restaurant phobic:

Situation: Entering restaurant and sitting down at table.

Physical feelings: 1 Rapid Relaxation in the taxi on my way to restaurant. 2 Active Relaxation while walking to table. 3 Make reservation to be sure of usual table by window. 4 Sit with back to restaurant so I can look out of the window.

Mental feelings: 1 Alistair's favourite subjects are: Golf/collecting antiques. Ask views about scandal in art world. 2 Remember his wife's birthday last Wednesday. 3 Ask about son's new job.

Positive Self-Talk: 'I know that I will get tense when we arrive at the restaurant but I will be able to cope effectively by following the advice on this card.'

Positive Self-Talk Statements and Cue Cards are powerful weapons in your fight against any type of phobia. Use them right from the start of your training and continue using them after the phobia has been defeated. They will help you perform more effectively no matter what activity is being carried out, reduce stress and sustain self-confidence.

Difficulty Three – The panic attack

As you work on this training programme, panic attacks will be less and less likely to occur. However, one may still strike 'out of the blue' and you must be prepared to cope with this event *without* resorting to avoidance. If possible, sit down or rest against a wall or tree. But do your best to remain in or near the place where the panic started.

Each letter in the word COPING stands for a point to bear in mind during and after the panic . . .

C – Comfort yourself with the knowledge that, although they may be painful and frightening, these feelings are perfectly natural and not in the least harmful. They do *not* mean that anything more dreadful will happen to you. Once the panic has passed it is unlikely to return for a considerable time.

O – Observe what is *actually* happening to your body instead of making matters worse by worrying about things which are never going to happen.

P – Practise relaxation. It will help you control the physical feelings associated with rising anxiety and may prevent the panic entirely. If the attack still occurs use relaxation immediately afterwards to dispel any remaining tension.

I – Imagine the pleasant scene which you envisaged at the end of your relaxation sessions.

N – Notice that when you stop fuelling your anxiety with negative thoughts your panic quickly subsides.

G – Go forward again in an easy and relaxed manner. Remember WASP.

Handling a panic attack in this positive manner will make it much easier for you to cope with similar anxiety in the future and so assist your training.

Remember . . . Very few people overcome their phobias without experiencing at least one set-back. Our feelings are variable and what was accomplished with relative ease one day may seem an almost insurmountable challenge the next.

If you suffered a panic attack and ran away before the fear subsided you may conclude that you are right back where you started. But this is not so. You have simply encountered a temporary obstacle. Continue with the programme and do not allow your confidence to be undermined.

Your training programme so far

At this point you should have had experience in all three methods of relaxation. You will have gathered quite a lot of information about your phobia in the Record Diary and should be working on a list of activities written out on the Progress Chart.

Each activity will be practised in fantasy on three separate occasions before attempting it in real life. Each activity will be such as to produce a slight amount of anxiety (about 4 on the rating scale).

During real life sessions you will use WASP and make use of comments written on Cue Cards. Should a panic attack occur you now know how to cope without allowing the experience to undermine your confidence. Each session must last at least fifteen minutes.

When an overall goal is reached it may be that your phobia has been defeated. It could also be that only one of the difficulties associated with a more complex phobic difficulty has been overcome. In this case you will want to construct a second Progress Chart and work in the same structured and methodical manner towards achieving overall goal number two. Continue in this way until there are no situations or activities left that you cannot cope with.

At the same time you will, of course, be doing a variety of other things not directly connected with the training. How you approach these activities can, however, still have a direct bearing on your success in this programme.

In Step Six I will explain how to tackle everyday challenges, and how to carry the progress you have made forward into your new life without fear.

You can read this section straight away and make use of the procedures I describe whenever they seem appropriate.

6

Living Without Fear

All programmes of change, whether these involve losing weight on a diet, building stamina through fitness training or learning to overcome acute anxiety, have two things in common. They are easier to start than to finish and more people begin them than complete them.

Fighting your phobia is no exception. The reasons for this loss of motivation are not hard to identify. As I explained in Part One, the efficiency of any form of learning depends on the type of rewards available. The more immediate and powerful these rewards the faster those lessons are mastered, and the stronger the motivation to continue.

We have seen that phobias arise because the rewards – a rapid reduction in distressing anxiety symptoms – provide just this type of instant, and intense, relief by avoiding a frightening situation.

When you attempt to make other significant changes in your lifestyle, however, the rewards are usually much less immediate. Consider dieters or joggers hoping to bring about physical improvements in the way they look or feel. Here the goal of a more shapely figure or better health can take weeks or even months. Meanwhile each is forced to follow a rather punishing way of life in order to attain those long-delayed goals. Chocolate bars, cream cakes and large helpings are forbidden. Physically tiring exercise must be taken in all weathers. Little wonder that, after a week or so, with the pointer on the bathroom scales showing little signs of a downward shift, and stamina hardly appearing to improve at all, both dieter and jogger find the immediate rewards of eating what they like and adopting a lazier way of living a more attractive option.

It will be the same with your own phobia-fighting programme. Over the next few weeks I am asking you to carry out regular practice sessions in a methodical and structured way. There will be times when you feel thoroughly bored with the whole thing and are tempted to give up – or at least postpone – the training. You'll start by telling yourself things like:

'I'm not in the mood today . . . I'll probably feel more enthusiastic tomorrow.'
'It's not convenient right now. I'll wait until next month.'

'Things are just not working out as I had hoped. I'll try another approach.'

There may also be occasions when, having come to a temporary halt for the reasons I explained in Step Five, you never manage to get going again. Almost anybody with a phobia which seriously restricts their lifestyle wants to enjoy freedom from fear. But many are really seeking some kind of 'miracle' treatment in which they can be a passive, rather than an active and involved, participant.

They feel there must be a 'pill' to take away their fears. There is no such medication. They sometimes believe that hypnosis might free them from anxiety. But all the research evidence shows that hypnosis makes no real or lasting difference in the majority of cases. They resort to acupuncture. Although valuable in some areas of physical therapy it has no effect on phobias.

That these approaches should fail is hardly suprising given what we now know about the phobic response. Once you have 'learned' something you do not unlearn it. To make changes you must learn an alternative way of behaving. This is the only option open to you.

Suppose that, having spoken English for twenty years you moved to a country where not a word of English was spoken. You would not try and 'unlearn' your English but to master the new language. At the start, because you were so familiar with English, using the new language would be difficult, slow, and frequently frustrating. You would probably be very tempted on occasions to give up and come home. In time, however, you would become equally fluent in the new vocabulary and wonder why you ever found it hard.

If you have been suffering from a phobia for many years then you will be extremely good at being a phobic. Where these fears are complex and place serious restrictions on you (such as agoraphobia and social phobia) it is virtually certain that much of your life will have been constructed around these fears. In order to live without such anxiety you must learn to do the things which your fears currently prevent.

If a phobia prevents you from travelling on a bus then you must learn to travel on buses without excessive anxiety. If a phobia prevents you from eating in public, giving a talk, expressing yourself in an interview, looking at birds or listening to thunder, then you must learn to do all these things. Only in this way will restrictions imposed by your phobia disappear. But it takes time, requires effort, and demands regular practice.

How to sustain your interest

To remain motivated you need to introduce deliberate rewards along the way. Of course your final reward will be the freedom achieved when the overall goal has been accomplished. But, since that will take some time to achieve you must give serious thought to ways of providing rewards at different stages of the programme.

The Progress Chart offers a minor source of rewards as you note each successful training session and watch the series of ticks marching triumphantly across the paper. Most people find Deep Relaxation pleasurable, so this too can become a source of enjoyment that maintains motivation.

But more tangible types of reward can also be used. Many people find it easier to keep going during a bad patch if they give themselves small rewards as different sub-goals are attained. For example you might decide to pay yourself a small amount for each tick on the chart. When a certain sum had been saved in this way the money can be spent on some enjoyable luxury – a magazine or a cinema ticket, a book, or a visit to the theatre. One of my clients saves to have a relaxing massage, another adds to his stamp collection, a third buys herself flowers, a fourth takes his partner to a restaurant.

If you decide to adopt this approach then decide in advance how much each training session is 'worth'. Immediately you have completed it and ticked the Progress Chart, make that payment to yourself. You need not necessarily do this in cash since what is called a 'Token Economy' is equally satisfactory. This means replacing real money with some sort of token – buttons or plastic counters for example. These tokens are stored in a special container which is kept somewhere prominent so that you can watch the 'savings' mount. When the time comes to pay yourself, the tokens are exchanged for real currency.

Another source of encouragement, especially if you have experienced a set-back, is the Record Diary. Glance back through its pages after working on the programme for a while and you will almost certainly be gratified at the goals achieved.

Your partner, family and friends also play an important part in sustaining motivation. Ask somebody close to you to read this book – especially the section directed at them – and to give active support to your programme of change.

Change in the long term

In addition to those activities included in the training schedule you will, of course, be continuing with your everyday life. It may well be that your phobia has gradually cut you off from friends, social activities and trips away from home which you once enjoyed. You may well have settled into a routine which centres on your house and family.

A crucial aspect of overcoming many phobias is to break out of this routine and develop interests away from home. You should begin to call on your neighbours, visit friends, organize outings, and join clubs. If your phobia has prevented you from working, then think seriously about trying to find a job. Even part-time work which takes you into a new environment will be helpful.

These are not activities to be put off to some time in the distant future but important ways of helping yourself right now. As well as offering you enjoyment and stimulation, they will provide an opportunity to practise going out and meeting people. By transforming trips away from home into interesting and rewarding activities in their own right you will have taken an essential step towards your new lifestyle.

Looking after your health

When depressed or anxious our appetite is affected and we find it difficult to take exercise. This combination of a poor diet and insufficient physical activity undermines emotional health, making us more vulnerable to emotional difficulties. In an earlier book* I described this as the 'Negative Fitness Cycle' and contrasted it to the 'Positive Fitness Cycle' in which physical and mental wellbeing build one upon the other to make us feel in peak condition. The important thing is to identify this downwards spiral and to realize that you can break free.

You can improve your general physical health as follows:

Diet: Eat well-balanced meals which include plenty of fresh fruit and vegetables, meat and fish. Include liver on the menu at least once a week as it is rich in many vitamins which combat stress. Vitamin B is especially helpful if you are constantly tense and you should consider a supplement or additional foods rich in this vita-

---

* FIT–KIT, Sheldon Press.

min. Wheat germ and brewers yeast mixed with milk is one source rich in B complex. In addition take one multivitamin tablet per day.

Try to eat a good breakfast which includes protein (egg, fish, meat) as well as carbohydrates. A high carbohydrate (cereal, toast, sugar) breakfast pours energy into the bloodstream in a short, sharp, burst). As a result any energy not used immediately is converted to fat. By mid-morning there is an energy crisis producing a feeling of weariness and, perhaps, depression.

When the first meal of the day includes both protein and carbohydrate, energy is released more slowly and over a longer period. In this way the mid-morning 'dip' is avoided. You will find it easier to eat a good breakfast if you do not have too much food last thing at night.

The large dinner makes no sense from a nutritional viewpoint since the only thing the body can do with energy released during sleep is to store it as fat. You wake up still full from the night before, eat very little before starting the day and so repeat the energy crisis cycle described above.

The golden rule of sensible eating is – breakfast like a king, lunch like a prince and sup like a pauper.

One final point – cut down on tea and coffee. Many anxious people drink six or more cups per day, often strong and black in the case of coffee. Caffeine is a powerful drug which arouses the nervous system and so lowers the threshold for anxiety. Reduce your intake to no more than three cups per day and avoid it within three hours of bedtime.

Exercise: The most effective form of exercise stimulates the heart and blood circulation (cardiovascular) system. Called aerobics, it need be neither time-consuming nor especially tiring.

What you should do is to *increase* your pulse rate by a specific amount and hold it at that new level for twelve minutes. How you raise your pulse is unimportant. On fine days you might like to go for a gentle jog in the park or in the country. On wet days you can equally well skip, run on the spot, or disco-dance to lively music indoors.

The key to success is to allow your body to tell you how hard to exercise – to let your heart guide the training schedule. Start by working out your personal overload heart rate – the extra work your heart must do during each twelve minute session.

You calculate the rate like this: 220 minus your age multiplied by the 'fitness factor', which is a number calculated according to your physical state. If you are in good physical shape your fitness factor is 0.8. If you are in moderate shape then it is 0.7. If you have not taken any exercise for quite a while and get breathless when climbing even a short flight of stairs then use a factor of 0.6.

Subtracting your age from 220 gives you the maximum heart overload. Multiplying it by the fitness factor tells you just how much faster your heart should be made to work during exercise. A couple of examples will make the method clear:

Peter is aged forty-five and in poor shape. Alison is thirty and in average condition.
How hard should each exercise?
Peter: fitness factor = 0.6
$220 - 45 \times 0.6 = 105$ beats per minute.

Alison: fitness factor = 0.6
$220 - 30 \times 0.7 = 133$ beats per minute.

To achieve a good level of fitness, Alison must therefore work harder than Peter. As his stamina improves, of course, he will need to work out at a higher pulse rate because his fitness factor will increase, first to 0.7 and then – if he continues to train – to 0.8. The same applies to Alison who could move from 133 beats per minute to a maximum of 152.

Read your heartbeats by counting the pulse in your wrist as follows: Rest the left wrist (palm upwards) in your right palm so that it lies between the thumb and forefinger. The tips of your third and fourth finger are now positioned over the pulse. Press gently. If you are unable to feel any pulse at first, move your fingers slightly. It will be detected as a throbbing beneath the finger tips. Count the number of beats in 15 seconds (use a digital read-out watch or one with a clear sweep second hand) and multiply by 4 to get the heart rate per minute.

When you first start exercising you should monitor your pulse rate every few minutes to make sure the heart is working neither too hard (more beats per minute than are needed) or not hard enough (fewer than the required number of beats per minute). With practice, however, you will find it quite easy to hold your heart rate at the desired level for the twelve minute exercise session.

As with any form of strenuous exercise it is advisable to check with your doctor before starting, if you are more than forty-five and out of shape, if you have high blood-pressure, a heart condition, are recuperating after a major operation, have diabetes or a serious illness.

Sleep: If you are not getting sufficient sleep, or that sleep is disturbed, then it becomes harder to shake off depression, control anxiety and build physical health. Here are some suggestions for overcoming insomnia.

1 Unwind for at least an hour prior to going to bed. Do not undertake any mentally stimulating activity. Watch an undemanding TV programme, listen to music or read something light and entertaining.

2 Carry out a session of Deep Relaxation prior to sleep.

3 Make up your mind that you will only lie in bed *not* sleeping, for a fixed amount of time – say fifteen to twenty minutes. If you are still awake at the end of this period get up and carry out some non-stimulating task, wash the dishes, read a magazine, and so on.

It does not matter what you do so long as you get out of bed first. This is because by lying there *not* sleeping you get into the habit of feeling more wide awake as soon as you slip between the sheets. In a fairly short space of time the bed can become a stimulus which prevents you from sleeping. The only way to prevent this is by training your body to link bed with sleep and little else.

4 Frequently a common obstacle to sleep is a seemingly endless succession of thoughts, ideas and problems chasing around and around in the brain. If this is a problem for you, the best way is to get out of bed and write them down. By bringing circling thoughts into the open you usually exorcise them – at least temporarily – from your mind.

5 Sleep is far harder to come by if you are physically tired. A twelve minute session of aerobic exercises during the day will help prepare your body for restful sleep.

Your life without fear

It is not easy to overcome a phobia which may have been your constant companion for years. But it is possible.

The procedures I have described have helped large numbers of phobic sufferers to rediscover the joy of living fully and freely as rulers of their own destiny rather than as slaves to distressing, painful and handicapping fears.

DAY ONE	DAY TWO	DAY THREE	DAY FOUR	DAY FIVE	DAY SIX	DAY SEVEN
DAYS 1–10 Procedure DEEP RELAXATION Two 20-minute sessions per day RECORD DIARY Keep a daily diary from now on until you have achieved all the goals you desire and your phobia has been overcome. Note anything you do which causes anxiety. As you start working through the list of sub-goals on your Progress Chart (during Steps Three and Four) include these in the Diary. PROGRESS CHART Identify an overall goal. Develop a list of sub-goals which will lead you towards this overall goal.						

Part Three

1
Timetable

This timetable offers only an approximate guide to the point at which new procedures should start. It should be modified to suit your particular needs. Do not worry if you progress slightly faster, or a little more slowly, than shown here. Pin it up prominently and write in each procedure as you start to work on it. Note, too, every training session, as this will help you to monitor your progress and check that no important points have been overlooked.

DAYS 1 – 10

Procedure

DEEP RELAXATION
Two 20-minute sessions per day

RECORD DIARY
Keep a daily diary from now on until you have achieved all the goals you desire and your phobia has been overcome.
   Note anything you do which causes anxiety. As you start working through the list of sub-goals on your Progress Chart (during Steps Three and Four) include these in the Diary.

PROGRESS CHART
Identify an overall goal. Develop a list of sub-goals which will lead you towards this overall goal.

DAYS 11 – 19

RAPID RELAXATION

Five or six sessions per day, each lasting about thirty seconds. You can use this in place of one DEEP RELAXATION session if you wish.

RECORD DIARY

Continue keeping notes under the seven headings.
Start developing Positive Self-Talk Statements and write these on your Cue Cards.

FANTASY TRAINING

One fifteen-minute session per day following Deep Relaxation. Start with first activity on your Progress Chart and work gradually up the list. Repeat each activity three times before moving to the next.

DAY EIGHT	DAY NINE	DAY TEN	DAY ELEVEN	DAY TWELVE	DAY THIRTEEN	DAY FOURTEEN
			DAYS 11–19 RAPID RELAXATION Five or six sessions per day, each lasting about 30 seconds. You can use this in place of one DEEP RELAXATION session if you wish. RECORD DIARY Continue keeping notes under the seven headings. Start developing Positive Self-Talk Statements and write these on your Cue Cards. FANTASY TRAINING One 15-minute session per day following Deep Relaxation. Start with first activity on your Progress Chart and work gradually up the list. Repeat each activity three times before moving to the next.			

DAYS 20 – 27

DEEP RELAXATION
One or two sessions per day as before.

RAPID RELAXATION
Several daily sessions. Use in real life before any stressful encounter or anxiety-arousing situation.

ACTIVE RELAXATION
Practise this after Deep Relaxation training. Use these skills in everyday situations as well.

FANTASY TRAINING
Continue working through your Progress Chart and ticking off each training session.

REAL LIFE TRAINING
After carrying out each activity three times in your imagination do the same thing in real life.

Remember WASP.

Use your Cue Cards and Positive Self-Talk Statements to help smooth your way.

Note training sessions on the Progress Chart and in your Record Diary.

Reward yourself for completing a certain number of sub-goals.

Be prepared to revise your training schedule to add or reduce the number of intermediate steps according to the progress made and any set-backs encountered.

Use COPING to help you deal with any panics.

Continue in this way until ALL your goals have been accomplished.

DAY FIFTEEN	DAY SIXTEEN	DAY SEVENTEEN	DAY EIGHTEEN	DAY NINETEEN	DAY TWENTY	DAY TWENTY-ONE
					DAYS 20–27 DEEP RELAXATION One or two sessions per day as before. RAPID RELAXATION Several daily sessions. Use in real life before any stressful encounter or anxiety-arousing situation. ACTIVE RELAXATION Practise this after Deep Relaxation training. Use these skills in everyday situations as well. FANTASY TRAINING Continue working through your Progress Chart and ticking off each training session. REAL LIFE TRAINING After carrying out each activity three times in your imagination do the same thing in real life.	

2
Record Diary

Rate your anxiety as follows:

Calm, confident and happy when carrying our activity 1

Slight apprehension but generally enjoyable 2

Neither anxiety nor pleasure obtained from activity 3

Some apprehension, manageable, but no pleasure 4

Very anxious and hard to remain in the situation 5

Attempt abandoned due to excessive anxiety 6

Keep notes of *any* relevant activities on a daily basis but identify training sessions with the letter (T).

Before I Start	What, When, Where?	Physical Feelings	Mental Feelings	What was good about the situation	Afterwards	Anxiety Rating

3

Progress Chart

Write your overall goal in the space at the left of the sheet and the sub-goals beneath it – starting with the easiest. Each activity should arouse slight but manageable anxiety. As you complete each training session tick it off on the Chart as shown in the illustration opposite. Here, simply to make the procedure clear, the ticks have been replaced by a small letter F indicating each Fantasy Session and a small letter R indicating activity carried out in Real Life.

PROGRESS CHART DATE STARTED:

Walk to bus stop alone and wait 5 minutes.	F	F	F	R	R	R																						
Ride one stop on bus and walk home on my own.				F	F	F	R	R	R																			
Ride one stop – Catch bus back home.							F	F	F	R	R	R																
Ride two stops and then bus back home.										F	F	F	R	R	R													
Bus into town centre and home.													F	F	F	R	R	R										
Bus into town – Wait 15 minutes – Come home.																F	F	F	R	R	R							
Bus to town, go into supermarket on quiet day – Home.																			F	F	F	R	R	R				
Shop at supermarket on busy day – Home.																						F	F	F	R	R	R	
TARGETS TO BE ACHIEVED: Remember — Carry out each one three times before proceeding.	1	2	3	4	5	6	7	1	2	3	4	5	6	7	1	2	3	4	5	6	7	1	2	3	4	5	6	7
	WEEK							WEEK							WEEK							WEEK						

PROGRESS CHART   **DATE STARTED:**

TARGETS TO BE ACHIEVED: Remember — Carry out each one three times before proceeding.	1 2 3 4 5 6 7 WEEK	1 2 3 4 5 6 7 WEEK	1 2 3 4 5 6 7 WEEK	1 2 3 4 5 6 7 WEEK

David Lewis has specially recorded a three cassette training course to accompany this book.

The first tape teaches you how to relax, deeply, quickly and easily under almost any circumstances. It also shows you how to create powerful mental images that allow you to carry out currently feared activities.

The second cassette describes how to 'manage' anxiety and explains how to develop a positive attitude towards your current problems.

The third, specialist tape, provides specific advice about ways of creating your own self-help training programme for a wide range of common phobias, including agoraphobia.

There are also tapes on overcoming depression, being more assertive, enhancing your social skills and coping with common problems of childhood.

For free information please write to:

Action on Phobias, 8 The Avenue, Eastbourne BN21 3YA.

Index

Overcoming Common Problems Series

For a full list of titles please contact
Sheldon Press, Marylebone Road, London NW1 4DU

Overcoming Common Problems Series

Everything You Need to Know about Shingles
DR ROBERT YOUNGSON

Everything You Need to Know about Your
Eyes
DR ROBERT YOUNGSON

Family First Aid and Emergency Handbook
DR ANDREW STANWAY

Feverfew
A traditional herbal remedy for migraine
and arthritis
DR STEWART JOHNSON

Fight Your Phobia and Win
DAVID LEWIS

Getting Along with People
DIANNE DOUBTFIRE

Getting Married
JOANNA MOORHEAD

Goodbye Backache
DR DAVID IMRIE WITH COLLEEN
DIMSON

Heart Attacks – Prevent and Survive
DR TOM SMITH

Helping Children Cope with Divorce
ROSEMARY WELLS

Helping Children Cope with Grief
ROSEMARY WELLS

Helping Children Cope with Stress
URSULA MARKHAM

Hold Your Head Up High
DR PAUL HAUCK

How to be a Successful Secretary
SUE DYSON AND STEPHEN HOARE

How to Be Your Own Best Friend
DR PAUL HAUCK

How to Control your Drinking
DRS W. MILLER AND R. MUNOZ

How to Cope with Stress
DR PETER TYRER

How to Cope with Tinnitus and Hearing
Loss
DR ROBERT YOUNGSON

How to Cope with Your Child's Allergies
DR PAUL CARSON

How to Cure Your Ulcer
ANNE CHARLISH AND DR BRIAN
GAZZARD

How to Do What You Want to Do
DR PAUL HAUCK

How to Get Things Done
ALISON HARDINGHAM

How to Improve Your Confidence
DR KENNETH HAMBLY

How to Interview and Be Interviewed
MICHELE BROWN AND GYLES
BRANDRETH

How to Love a Difficult Man
NANCY GOOD

How to Love and be Loved
DR PAUL HAUCK

How to Make Successful Decisions
ALISON HARDINGHAM

How to Move House Successfully
ANNE CHARLISH

How to Pass Your Driving Test
DONALD RIDLAND

How to Say No to Alcohol
KEITH McNEILL

How to Spot Your Child's Potential
CECILE DROUIN AND ALAIN DUBOS

How to Stand up for Yourself
DR PAUL HAUCK

How to Start a Conversation and Make
Friends
DON GABOR

How to Stop Smoking
GEORGE TARGET

How to Stop Taking Tranquillisers
DR PETER TYRER

How to Stop Worrying
DR FRANK TALLIS

How to Study Successfully
MICHELE BROWN